Word Rounds

A history of words, both medical and non-medical
and their relationship to one another.

by

AF597444

Barton J. Gershen, MD

Flower Valley Press
Gaithersburg, Maryland

Copyright © 1999 by Barton J. Gershen

All rights reserved. No part of this book may be reproduced or electronically stored in any form without the written permission of Flower Valley Press.

ISBN – 1-886388-16-4

Library of Congress Cataloging in Publication Data

Gershen, Barton J.

Word Rounds: a history of words, both medical and nonmedical,
and their relationship to one another / Barton J. Gershen.
p. cm.
Includes bibliographical references and index.
ISBN 1-886388-16-4
1. Medicine—Terminology. 2. English language—Etymology
3. English language—Medical English. I. Title.

[R123 .G46 2000]
610'.1'4—dc21
99-058919

Printed in the United States of America

10 9 8 7 6 5 4 3 2 1

www.WordRounds.com

Flower Valley Press
7851 C Beechcraft Ave.
Gaithersburg, MD 20879
301-654-1996

Dedication

To Enid

Without you there are no words.

Introduction

I am not an English authority, semanticist, or etymologist. My profession is that of a physician, internist, and clinical cardiologist – yet I have been fascinated by words, especially their origins, since I was quite young. Actually, I remember well the origin of this enchantment.

I was a freshman undergraduate student at the University of Vermont. The year was 1950, and I sat rather bored in an English class, one required by the premedical curriculum. The professor, a rather corpulent, unkempt character, stood eyeing us warily, quite cognizant of our collective apathy. After all, he knew that most of us planned a career in medicine, or some other scientific discipline. What possible use would a course in English afford us? Besides, we had all sat through several years of English classes at our respective high schools. What could he teach us that was new and useful?

And then, in a reedy, rather nasal voice, he began the story of Martin of Tours, a child born in the third century AD. Martin's father was a soldier in the Roman Legion, and when he grew to manhood, Martin, too, joined the army. One winter's day, as his regiment entered the gates to the walled city of Amien, Martin spied a beggar sitting on a snowdrift, just outside the gate. The man was starving and freezing to death. Martin reigned in his steed, leaped off, removed his heavy woolen cape, tore it in half, and placed it around the beggar's shoulders. Then, with the remaining half-cape about his own shoulders, Martin mounted his horse and rode on into the city.

Shortly afterward, Martin left the Roman Legion and entered a monastery. He later was appointed bishop of Tours and founded the first monastery in Gaul (modern day France). After his death he was canonized, and has since become the patron saint of France.

His half cape became a sacred relic, and was carried into battle by Frankish kings, to ensure success in combat. During peacetime the sacred object was maintained in a special consecrated room within the king's palace. The latin word for **cape** is *cappa*, deriving from the fact that it had a head covering, or hood, and the term for head was *caput*. A small cape (or half-cape) was known as a *capella*, and eventually the room which housed St. Martin's cape also became known as the *capella*.

A custodian was appointed to guard the famous relic. This man was one of the palace monks, and became known as the *capellanus*. Eventually, the room (the *capella*) became known as the *chapele,* as Latin evolved into French. And the *capellanus* became the *chapelain.* In English, of course, they became the chaplain and the chapel.

Choir practice was usually conducted in that hallowed Cape room, and – since there was no musical accompaniment – this form of singing became known as chanting "in the manner of the chapel" – *a capella.*

For me, a moment of intellectual epiphany had occurred, as I realized that words had origins and memoirs. I have never forgotten this modest little English professor, nor the impact he had on my life. Since then, although medicine has been my metier, my avocation has been word histories.

For sixteen years I have written a column on words, most of which have had medical appeal. These have been published in **Montgomery Medicine** and the **Maryland Medical Journal**, and this book represents a collection of some of those essays. I wish to thank the editors and editorial boards of each of those journals for permission to reprint many of my original articles.

Further acknowledgements must go to the following superb references, all of which have contributed to this volume:

American Heritage Dictionary
Asimov,Isaac *Biographical Encyclopedia of Science and Technology*
Asimov, Isaac *Words of Science*
Ayto, Arcade *Dictionary of Word Origins*
Barnhart, *Dictionary of Etymology*
Brewer's Dictionary of Phrase and Fable
Brewer's Dictionary of Twentieth-Century Phrase and Fable
Choate, *The Dictionary of American Bird Names*
Ciardi, *A Browser's Dictionary*
Ciardi, *A Second Browser's Dictionary*
Ciardi, *Good Words To You*
Danner and Noel, *Academic Vocabulary*
Dirckx, *The Language of Medicine*
Dorland, *Illustrated Medical Dictionary*
Encyclopedia Brittanica
Espy, *Thou Improper, Thou Uncommon Noun*
Firkin and Whitworth, *Dictionary of Medical Eponyms*, 2nd Edition

Flavell, *Dictionary of Word Origins*
Funk, *A Hog On Ice*
Funk, *Heavens to Betsy*!
Funk, *Horsefeathers*
Funk, *Thereby Hangs a Tale*
Harder, *Illustrated Dictionary of Place Names*
Haubrich, *Medical Meanings, A Glossary of Word Origins*
Hendrickson, *The Dictionary of Eponyms*
Holt, Henry *Encyclopedia of Word and Phrase Origins*
Kass, *Perfecting the World: the Life and Times of Thomas Hodgkin*
Larouse, *Biographical Dictionary*
Lifton, *The Nazi Doctors*
Lourie, *Medical Eponyms*: *Who Was Coude'*
Magalini and Scrascia *Dictionary of Medical Syndromes*, 2nd Edition
Maleska, *A Pleasure in Words*
McGrew, *Encyclopedia of Medical History*
Morris, *Dictionary of Word and Phrase Origins*
NTC's *Dictionary of Latin and Greek Origins*
Rose, *Curator of the Dead: Thomas Hodgkin (1798-1866)*
Rosenfeld, *Thomas Hodgkin: Morbid Anatomist & Social Activist*
Partridge, *Origins A Short* Etymological *Dictionary of Modern English*
Shipley, *Dictionary of Word Origins*
Snyder, *Encyclopedia of the Third Reich*
Stedman, *Medical Dictionary*
Stewart, *American Place Names*
Trager, *The People's Chronology*
Webster's *New Biographical Dictionary*
Webster's *New World Dictionary, 3rd Edition*
Webster's *Word Histories*

Inadvertent Omissions:
Flexner, *I Hear America Talking*
Flexner, *Listening to America*

Contents

Medical Patois

Three weeks into my freshman year in medical school my mother had the entire family over for brunch. Proudly she turned to her only child and in the most accomplished stage whisper said: "Say something in medicine for us." My cheeks flaming, I controlled the vitriolic urge to respond by naming some indelicate perineal organ. Instead, entirely out of character, I reticently stammered some self-conscious apology and demurred.

Of course there had been a jot of humor in my mother's request. And more than an iota of implicit truth.

The truth is that our fraternity does speak a foreign tongue. We converse in an idiom filled with scientific Greek and Latin roots, sobriquets, eponyms, acronyms, and other diminutives - all peculiar to our professional order. It is an exotic jargon, scholarly and precise, but often alien to other members of society, and filled with elements of enchantment, dread, and mystery.

In fact it often is alien to us - its very speakers. As medical neophytes we are unceremoniously dumped into a unique world without a clue about its history, or the origin of its terminology. The truth of a word (Greek *etymon*) is implied by its **etymology**. Word histories, the derivation of terms, tells us something about what those words mean and how they got to mean it. In this volume, I share with you some of those truths that have delighted and stimulated me, the eccentricities of our medical dialect, as well as some non-medical terms that I have found fascinating.

Anatomy is a good place to start. The **mastoid**, that smooth, spherical outcropping of the temporal bone located behind the ear, received its name from some extremely imaginative, if somewhat lecherous, ancient prosector. He thought it looked like a tiny breast (Greek: *mastos*: "breast" + *oides*: "like").

The **Duodenum**, the first section of the small intestine, was named for its length. It is roughly twelve finger widths long (Latin - *duodecim*: "twelve", which, in turn, is from Latin *duo*: "two" + *decem*: "ten". [December was originally the tenth month of the Roman calendar, just as September was the seventh (*septem*: "seven"), October the eighth (*octo*: "eight"), and November ninth (*novem*: "nine"). Julius and Augustus Caesar in a frenzy of narcissism, borrowed some days from the other months and stuffed two months in between June and September - thus totally obscuring the etymology of the last four months of each year.]

Arteries are also inaccurately named. The word stems from Greek *arteria* which originates from *aer*: "air" + *tereo*: "to keep", that is something which holds air or acts as an air duct. At necropsy, most arteries are found to be empty. To the early anatomists they appeared to carry air, and were therefore called "air keepers". (The **Jejunum** is also empty at most dissections. Thus, Latin - *jejunus*: "empty" or "hungry". Do you remember a delicious pomposity from Woodie Allen's "Annie Hall": "You are so **jejune**!")

The names of two arteries are especially intriguing. In ancient Greece, charlatans attracted an audience by paralyzing a goat with their hands. They pressed firmly on arteries within the goat's neck and it promptly fell unconscious. The Greek word *karotikos* means "to stun or render unconscious", and thus the **Carotid** arteries were named.

The legend of the second artery begins with the famous Roman physician Galen. Born in 130 A.D. in Pergamum, Asia Minor (now Bergama, a town in western Turkey), he became physician to the gladiators in Rome. His reputation soon spread and he became the preeminent physician in the city, attending three emperors. He was the first to recognize that arteries contained blood not air and, although he had never performed a dissection, his anatomic drawing were regarded as the quintessence of truth and perfection.

1400 years later they were still venerated with the respect accorded divine revelation. (Medicine had its Dark Ages along with the rest of civilization.) Then, Andreas Vesalius was born. He, too, perused the works of the renowned Galen. But in Italy, where he had journeyed following graduation from Montpellier and Paris, physicians were actually performing dissections! Vesalius, therefore, had the opportunity to verify the accuracy of Galen's work, some of which he found to be quite imprecise. Nevertheless, in his classic and monumental treatise on the anatomy of the human body - *De Humani Corporis Fabrica*, Vesalius employed most of Galen's anatomic terms.

In an illustration of the arteries originating from the aortic arch, Galen had inadvertently failed to label one of the principal vessels. Since he found no name with which to identify the artery, Vesalius - perhaps in a facetious spirit - called it "the anonymous" or "un-named" vessel. In Latin this is known as the *arteria innominata* - the Innominate artery.

Some anatomic structures were originally named for their resemblance to other objects (as with the breast and mastoid bone). The

Coronary Arteries encircle the heart like a crown, the Latin for which is *corona*. And the **Mitral valve**, with its bicuspid leaflets, looked to some devout anatomist like the twin peaks of a Bishop's **miter** - the tall hat worn by the Pope and his bishops. The **Coccyx** reminded some prosector, who was an avid bird watcher, of the Cuckoo's beak. The Greek word for Cuckoo is *kokkyx*.

The Greek word for crow is *korax* - someone else imagined the **coracoid** process resembled a crow's beak.

Then there are the eponymous structures - those which began life as proper names - only to be lower-cased by history. **Gabriele Fallopio** initiated his career as a canon of the cathedral at Modena. Fortunately for us, Fallopio converted to medicine and became the most distinguished of the 16th century Italian anatomists. He was Vesalius' favorite pupil and succeeded him as Professor of Surgery and Anatomy at the University of Padua. Fallopio described the 5th, 8th, and 9th cranial nerves, the Chorda Tympani, the placenta, vagina, the cochlea of the inner ear, and the oviducts which bear his name - the **fallopian tubes**.

A contemporary and rival of Fallopio was **Bartolomeo Eustachi**, physician to Pope Julius III, and Professor of Anatomy at the Collegio delle Sapienze in Rome. He described the adrenal glands, the 6th cranial nerve, and the thoracic duct, in addition to the tiny tubes that connect the middle ear with the pharynx - the **eustachian tubes**. These were named in Eustachi's honor over a century after his death by a man named **Antonio Maria Valsalva**. (The **Valsalva maneuver** - forced expiration against a closed glottis - was introduced as a test for middle ear infections in 1704.)

To return for a moment to the Greek word *mastos* : "breast" (as in **mastectomy**, **mastitis** and **mastoid**), it is fascinating to note that the Greeks also used two other terms to designate that captivating organ - *mazos* and *mamme*. The latter word was borrowed by the Romans and altered to Latin *mammae* from which stem **mammary** and **mammal** (animals which suckle their young). However, insofar as I can ascertain, there exists only one word that derives from the Greek word *mazos*.

That word was used to denote a mythological tribe of women who lived in Scythia near the Black Sea. (The region known as Scythia is now the Crimean region of southern Ukraine. In the 4th century B.C. a tribe of fierce, nomadic, female warriors from Iran, were said to have settled in this region and were known as Scythians.) The women were skilled archers who - in order to draw their bowstrings further back, - cut off their right breasts. These mythological females were therefore known as *a*:"without" + *mazos*:"breast" - **Amazons.**

There is a further, curious twist to this story. In 1543, after participating with **Pizzaro** in the conquest of Peru, a Spanish explorer named **Francisco de Orellana** decided to explore the unknown waters of the Maranon River east of Quito. Drifting along with the current he mapped the entire river to its mouth. But along the way he claimed to have been attacked by a fierce tribe of female warriors. Orellana insisted that these were muscular women who each lacked one breast. He believed that he had discovered the mythological **Amazons**.

Despite the manifest absurdity of this claim, Orellana had suddenly renamed the Maranon River. It is now called the **Amazon River**. From a Greek breast, through a mythical tribe of female warriors, to the second longest river in the world - such is the odyssey of some words, and the fascination of etymology.

Anatomy Lesson

It was the year that ended the tragedy in Korea. Peace was confirmed by signatures on a contract written in a quaint village named Panmunjon, while Marilyn's magnificence was flawlessly displayed in the centerfold of a new magazine, published by a man named Hefner. And the Rosenbergs were executed in the electric chair.

I was 20 years old and stood very quietly behind a bookshelf in the shadowy corner of the anatomy lab. There were fifteen dissecting tables. On each, beneath a dark cover, lay a cadaver whose human outline was thinly veiled by its forbidding mantle.

It was the first day of the first week of my first year in medical school, and we were being introduced to our silent companions for the first time. Images of Frankenstein, the Wolf man, Dracula, and the Mummy - Lon Chaney, Jr., Boris Karloff, and Bela Lugosi - whirled incessantly in my head.

It was my first anatomy class, and my medical career almost ended that day. I often think about those classes, days of terror - and perplexity. Let me share with you, as well, some of its terminology.

Many early **prosectors** had named parts of the body for objects which they seemed to resemble.(Latin: *prosectus* past participle of the Latin verb *prosecare* - "to cut before". The root *secare* - "to cut" - can be found in the geometric term **secant** - a line which is **bisected**. *Secare* is present, as well, at an **intersection** - a street "cut into" by another.)

The imagination of anatomists is boundless. The **deltoid** muscle is somewhat triangular, resembling the fourth letter of the Greek alphabet - *delta* + *oides* : "like" - that is, "like a delta". (The delta of a river is also named for that Greek letter, since it, too, resembles a triangle.)

In a comparable simile, the **trapezius** is named for its resemblance to a trapezoid.(Greek *tetra*: "four" + *peza*: "foot" -that is, "having four feet" - a reference to a small square bench or table.) Likewise, the **coracoid** process, a bony, scapular nubbin from which arises the short head of the Biceps and the Coraco-brachialis muscle, looked like a crow's beak to some ancient dissector. (Greek *korakoeides* : "like a raven").

The **coccyx** also resembled a bird (from Greek *kokkux:* "a cuckoo") since it was shaped like a cuckoo's beak. A forearm bone, the **radius,** was directly from Latin: "the spoke of a wheel" - which, of course, is also what one inscribes when you draw a line from the center of a circle to its edge.

Aristotle named the **phalanges** (*phalanx* : "digit") because they reminded him of the military formations used by the Greeks, and Romans. (A Greek *phalanx* consisted of heavily armed infantrymen standing shoulder to shoulder in files, generally eight men deep.) The Latin word for a finger or toe is *digitus*, which leads directly to the English **digit**. The term "digit" when employed to indicate a number stems directly from the aboriginal convention of counting on one's fingers.

The **xiphoid** process derives from its shape - Greek *xiphos*: "sword"+ *eidos*: "like". The Romans called it the **ensiform** process - Latin *ensis*: "sword" + *forma*: "form". The **duodenum**, on the other hand, was not named for its resemblance to anything. It was simply twelve fingers in length - Latin *duodecim*: "twelve" (two plus ten). In German the duodenum is *der zwelffingerdarm.*

The **sacrum** was called the *os sacrum* by the Romans - the "sacred bone". The Greeks before them, also had believed the bone was holy, calling it *hieron ostoun*. This was probably because the sacrum - the last bone to decay in a rotting corpse - made it the likely bone around which a new body might be constructed in the afterlife.

At the opposite end of the body sits the *calvaria*, Latin for "the roof of the skull". Outside the city gates of ancient Jerusalem there stood a forbidding hill, whose baleful and portentous shape suggested a skull, to prehistoric Palestinians. In Aramaic the hill was called **Golgotha**: "skull hill". In Latin it was known as ***Calvary***, the site of Christ's crucifixion.

Finally, we come to the Latin word *cubitum*:"the elbow". A unit of ancient measure, the **cubit**, derives from it. One cubit is roughly the distance from the tip of the third finger to the elbow, about 20 inches. The hollow space "in front of the elbow", the **antecubital fossa**, is self-explanatory. However, things become a little more interesting when one remembers how the elite Romans ate their meals. They usually reclined as they gorged. To do this they had to lean on their elbows for support. The idea of "lying down", soon became inextricably linked with the word for elbow. Thus we have **incubate**: "to lie on", and **decubitus**: "from lying down" (the proximate cause of **decubitus ulcers**). In addition, we have **concubine**, (Latin *com*: "with" + *cubare* "to lie down") a subtle pejorative clearly fulfilling the etymologic definition.

We also have those gargoyles of Freudian Eolithic fiction, the **incubi** (Latin in: "upon" + cubare, that is, "to lie down upon".) and the **succubi** (Latin sub: "under" + cubare, that is, "to lie down under").

Gremlins don't hold a candle to them. The incubus, an evil male spirit, violated tender young women as they slept. Not to be outdone, the succubus was a wicked female apparition, who forced herself under innocent males.

Oh, to sleep, perchance to dream...

The Quaker and the Jew

The year was 1798. Napoleon Bonaparte, a Frenchman, was designing a treacherous coup d'etat - while Edward Jenner, an Englishman, was about to publish an "Inquiry into the Causes and Effects of the Variolae Vaccinae". King George III sat despotically on his British throne, while his former colonists in democratic America were about to pass the Alien and Sedition Acts.

On August 17th of that year, in the village of Pentonville eight miles north of London, a child was born to a devout Quaker family. They named him Thomas. The parents, John and Elizabeth, were quite skeptical of ever having children, for their first two sons had died in infancy. This child, however, was sturdy and full of energy.[1]

Their home was cheerful and sunny, despite the overwhelming prejudice that often pursues those who dress or speak peculiarly. And Thomas certainly experienced social ostracism because of his orthodox Quaker manner. But this bigotry never dissuaded him from his firm belief in the equality of all people.

When he was 20 Thomas wrote "An Essay on the Promotion of Civilization" in which he said, "my life's aim will be to protect the primitive aboriginal people of all continents of the world to which European traders are moving". He pledged to devote his life to that admirable end. He abhorred slavery and helped found the British Aborigine Society, dedicated to those humanitarian purposes. He reached adulthood nurtured by these beliefs, quite confident in his own ability to correct the evils of an arrogant, uncaring society.

Thomas was quite short and rather awkward. Nevertheless, he soon discovered that his values were ardently supported by Sarah Goodly, an attractive second cousin. The two soon fell in love, and Thomas asked for her hand - but the elders of the church refused to permit the marriage.

The couple was devastated. There was a poignant farewell, and a dejected Thomas left Pentonville for St. Thomas and Guy's Hospital in London, to begin his education in medicine. There he was soon recognized as a bright, promising scholar and in 1820 he was promoted to the medical school at Edinburgh University.

In 1821 he traveled to France and spent the year as a student with Rene Laennac at the Charite Hospital in Paris. Laennac had just invented the monaural wooden stethoscope and Thomas quickly learned the new art of mediate auscultation. On October 5,1822, having returned from his sabbatical in France, Thomas presented a paper at Guy's Hospital on the principles of stethoscopy. His lecture was met with indifference by many. However, William Stroud was so impressed that he soon developed the flexible monaural stethoscope. (One should not be too surprised at the tepid response that attended Laennac's innovative device. In the first American edition of Laennac's *Treatise on the Diseases of the Chest*, John Forbes, M.D. prefaced the book as follows: "That it will ever come into general use, notwithstanding its value, I am extremely doubtful, because its beneficial application requires much time and gives a good bit of trouble both to the patient and the practitioner.......It must be confessed that there is something even ludicrous in the picture of a grave physician proudly listening through a long tube applied to the patient's thorax,as if the disease were a living being that could communicate its condition ....")

In 1828 Thomas published a short paper in the Medical Gazette of London entitled "On Retroversion of the Valves of the Aorta", in which he first described a musical "purring, thrilling or sawing kind of noise" in association with retroversion of an aortic cusp. He termed it the *bruit de scie* and it is sometimes eponymously associated with his name.

Shortly thereafter Thomas was appointed director of Pathology at Guy's Hospital. Officially, this title was known as "Curator of the Dead". There he spent the next fifteen years meticulously conducting autopsies and joyfully teaching on ward rounds. The students loved him - voting him unanimously as their favorite instructor.

It was about this time in his life that Thomas met an influential Jewish family. They became private patients of his and their oldest son Moses soon became his best friend. They were originally silk merchants from Spain, and had immigrated with their wealth to England. Once established in London, Moses and his brother had applied for - and received - a seat on the illustrious London Stock Exchange. They were the first Jews approved for that influential position.

Soon Moses had augmented his original fortune several times. He then married into the Rothschild family, the renowned banking moguls, and at age forty retired to devote his energy and huge resources to public and private charities. He was an Orthodox Jew and donated much of his opulence to building schools and hospitals and founding agricultural settlements in Palestine.He was appointed Sheriff of London and, in 1837,was knighted by Queen Victoria.

Thomas, too, was accomplishing some important goals. In 1832 The Journal of the Medical and Chirurgical Society of London published his paper on "Some Morbid Appearances of the Adsorbent Glands and Spleen" which received favorable critical acclaim.

And then came the catastrophic event that would end his career.

Dr. James Chomley, medical director of Guy's Hospital (officially termed "Physician to Guy's Hospital") suddenly died, and on Wednesday, the 6th of September 1837, twenty-six members of the Board of Directors of Guy's Hospital met to vote for a successor. The Board unanimously voted for Dr. Thomas Addison (famed for "Addison's Disease") to replace him. They next had to vote on someone to fill the post of "Assistant Physician to Guy's Hospital", which had been vacated by Addison.

There were officially seven candidates, however, everyone connected with the hospital knew that only two names were to be considered at that meeting. One was Dr.Benjamin Babington whose sister was married to Richard Bright ("Bright's Disease"), and whose father had previously been an admired and respected Physician to Guy's, from 1795-1811. The second major candidate was the "Curator of the Dead", the Quaker physician Thomas.

The hospital treasurer spoke first and was vehement in his opposition to Thomas, specifically because of his leadership in the Aborigine Society. Thomas received only two votes, and Benjamin Babington became the new Assistant Physician to Guy's Hospital.

The popular "Curator of the Dead" immediately resigned in anger. He never again set foot in Guy's Hospital - or taught another student. Or wrote another medical paper.

Moses took his disconsolate friend away. They made several philanthropic trips to the European contininent and to the Mid East.

In the spring of 1866 Thomas made his last journey. A severe locust infestation in Palestine had decimated that year's crops. Moses and Thomas travelled there to see if they could somehow assist the starving population.

Thomas was not feeling well when they left, and by the time they had arrived in Alexandria, Egypt, he fell gravely ill and could go no further. He remained with the British Consular agent and was attended by a Dr. Socci, an Egyptian physician.

On April 4,1866 at 5:15 P.M. Thomas died of dysentery.

His anguished friend Moses wrote: "It has pleased the All Mighty to take him from us...one so guileless, so pious, so amiable in his private life...so respected in his public career, and so desirous to assist with all his heart in the amelioration of the condition of the Human race."

Thomas was buried in a small cemetery in Jaffa near the Tabatha Girl's School.

A grieving Moses had an obelisk erected before the grave. It says simply:

> "Here rests the body of **Thomas Hodgkin**, M.D, of Bedford Square, London."

The grave is never overgrown with weeds, for it is perpetually attended by the residents of Jaffa – few of whom know anything about the man whose last resting place they attend.

Hodgkin's name, of course, has been bequeathed to medical posterity for his original description of the disease which bears it. His initial report was based strictly on gross anatomic description of the six cases examined by him at Guy's Hospital. (Microscopes were available to physicians of that era, however, they were used only to explore liquid specimens. The microtome, an instrument capable of slicing solid tissue into sections thin enough to be viewed by the microscopist, was not invented by Schwann until 1838 - after Hodgkin had left Guy's Hospital.)

In 1926 Herbert Fox, a New York pathologist, microscopically re-examined the tissue specimens from which Hodgkin had reached his conclusions. He reported that one was actually tuberculosis, a second syphilis, and a third was a non-Hodgkin's Lymphoma.Only three of the original specimens actually represented "Hodgkin's Disease".

Moses died twenty years after Hodgkin.His full name was Sir Moses Haim Montefiore, and there is a monument to him as well.

It may be seen in the Bronx, New York.

It's called **Montefiore Hospital**.

(1. See references Kass; Rose; and Rosenfeld.)

Eponyms I

The majority of medical eponyms are easily identifiable, for example, **Bright's** Disease, or **Raynaud's** Syndrome. For the uninitiated, Bright's Disease is a kidney disorder, which is also known as glomerulonephritis. It usually occurs in children and results from an infection with certain streptococcal bacteria. **Richard Bright** was a colleague of **Thomas Addison** and **Thomas Hodgkin**, at Guy's Hospital in London. He described the renal disorder that bears his name, in 1836. Ironically, of the three preserved kidney specimens from his original index cases, two were recently shown to have been due to membrano-proliferative glomerulonephritis, and the third was a result of amyloidosis of the kidneys, rather than acute glomerulonephritis.

Raynaud's Syndrome describes the remarkable color changes that occur in the fingers of certain patients, on exposure to cold temperature or chilly objects. The digits become white, then blue (and painful), and finally bright red. This disorder was first described by **Maurice Raynaud** in 1862.

However, there are numerous eponymic syndromes that are not so easily identified. For instance **brownian** motion, which describes the incessant, random microscopic movement of particles in suspension. It was first noticed in 1827 by **Robert Brown**, a botanist and physician, while observing pollen grains floating in water. This phenomenon was so fascinating that it ultimately engaged the attention of **Albert Einstein**. In a 1905 paper, he demonstrated that it was the infinitesimal pressure exerted by surrounding water molecules bumping into the pollen grains, which caused them to wobble. Incidentally, Robert Brown was the first scientist to publish a work on the flora of Australia, the first to distinguish between gymnosperms and angiosperms in botany, and the first to describe and name the nucleus of the cell.

Gymnosperms are plants - such as conifers - whose seeds are naked, that is, not enclosed within an ovary. The term is from Greek *gumnos*: "naked" and *sperma*: "seed". The word **gymnasium** derives from Greek gumnos through gumnazein: "to exercise naked", a commonpractice in ancient Greece. Indeed, Greek wrestling was practiced in the nude, a behavior that seems quite curious to us today.

Angiosperms are plants whose seeds are contained within an ovary. From Greek *angos*: "a vessel". **Angiograms** are radiographic images of blood vessels (Greek *graphein*: "to write"), and **angioplasty** is the technique by which stenotic arteries are enlarged through inflation of a tiny balloon on the tip of a catheter (Greek *plassein*: "to mold". The word **plastic** derives from the same Greek source.)

The **Golgi** complex or apparatus, is a cytoplasmic organelle, which lies near the cell nucleus, manufactures lysosome, and stores hormones within its secretory granules. It is named for **Camillo Golgi** an Italian histologist. Golgi also developed the silver nitrate method of staining nerve cells (now called Golgi cells), which ultimately led to the birth of a new medical specialty: neurology.

Milkman's Syndrome, spontaneous, symmetrical pseudofractures, was reported in 1930 by a radiologist from Scranton, Pennsylvania - **Louis Arthur Milkman**. The syndrome had actually been first described by a Swiss physician, **Emil Looser**, therefore, the lesions are occasionally referred to as **Looser Zones**.

Baker's Cyst - like Milkman's Syndrome - is totally unrelated to the food industry. The disorder is named for **William Morrant Baker**, an English surgeon who operated at St. Bartholomew's Hospital, and for many years was **Sir James Paget's** assistant. Baker described the syndrome of herniated popliteal bursa in 1877. (Paget is familiar to us because of the boney disorder - osteitis deformans - which he described in 1877. He also described an eczematoid lesion of the nipples, occasionally seen in ductal carcinoma.) St. Bartholomew's Hospital is named for Saint Bartholomew, one of the Twelve Apostles. The name means "son of Tolmai", deriving from Hebrew *bar*: "son of". Those who work there affectionately know the hospital as "St. Bart's". (Incidentally, **Bart's Hemoglobin**, an abnormal hemoglobin having four gamma chains, is named for St. Bartholomew's Hospital where it was first detected.)

Negri bodies are not black. They are spherical or ovoid eosinophilic inclusions, which are located within the cytoplasm of nerve cells. These inclusion bodies are pathognomonic of rabies, and were first observed in 1903 by **Adelchi Negri**, an Italian physician. Negri had been Golgi's assistant, but quickly rose to full professor of bacteriology at the University of Pavi. His research material consisted of dogs, rabbits, and cats which had been infected with a street virus, a few lab-infected animals, and one human - a 64 year old woman who had died of a rabid dog bite. Unfortunately, science did not have this gifted investigator very long. Six years after marrying his colleague Lina Luzzani, Negri died of pulmonary tuberculosis at age 36.

Bacteria are characterized by **gram** positive or gram negative staining. The technique was discovered by **Hans Christian Joachim Gram**, a postgraduate student working with **Carl Friedlander**. One morning Gram accidentally spilled Lugol's iodine solution over a bacterial slide. In attempting to wash it off with alcohol, Gram made his momentous discovery. (Incidentally, **Lugol**'s solution, a mixture of 5% Iodine plus 10% potassium Iodide, was initially used to treat pulmonary tuberculosis by **Jean Guillaume Auguste Lugol**. It was not found to be useful, but was thereafter effectively applied to the treatment of thyrotoxicosis by **Henry Stanley Plummer**, a physician at the Mayo Clinic. Plummer, of course, had nothing to do with Watergate. He was half the team of **Plummer - Vinson**, whose syndrome consists of dysphagia and glossitis and is found in iron deficient, middle-aged women.

In 1951, Dr. George Gey of Johns Hopkins University established a cell culture from a patient with cervical carcinoma. Today, descendants of that cell line may be found in laboratories all over the world. They are used as a viral culture medium, and are known as **hela cells** - an acronym for the patient from whom they were initially derived - **Helen Lacks**.

In 1943, a young girl named **Margaret Tracy** fractured her leg. It was a severe compound fracture, which understandably became infected. Cultures taken from the wound grew a gram positive, spore-forming rod. A polypeptide was isolated from the organism and discovered to be, curiously and almost improbably, an antimicrobial substance. The bacteria, which had produced this biological paradox, was *Bacillus subtilis*. It became known as the Tracy I strain in honor of its immediate host (or hostess), and the antibiotic, which was derived from that culture, was logically named **Bacitracin**.

Other patients have contributed their names to eponymic history. In 1952, Dr. Rosemary Biggs and her associates from Oxford, England reported a new hemorrhagic disorder. It resembled classic hemophilia, and was also an autosomal, sex-linked recessive illness. The description was published in **The British Medical Journal** under the title:"*Christmas Disease: A Condition Previously Mistaken for Haemophilia.*" The etiology of this genetic illness is currently understood to be a deficiency of factor IX. The disease itself was named for the youngest patient in Dr. Biggs series of seven cases: **Stephen Christmas**.

In the same way, factor XII was named **Hageman** Factor and factor X **Stuart-Prower** Factor - each for patients with the specific deficiency. **Friedlander**, mentioned above, deserves some recognition for the bacterium he described in 1882, **Friedlander's bacillus**. Today we refer to it as *Klebsiella pneumoniae*. Its genus name is derived from another outstanding bacteriologist, **Theodor Albrecht Edwin Klebs**, who is also remembered for his discovery (with **Friederich Loeffler**) of the **Klebs-Loeffler** bacillus, *Corynebacterium diphtheriae*. (Greek *koryne*: "club" + *bakterion*: "little rod", i.e. club-shaped rods, and Greek *dipthera*: "membrane" - referring to the pseudomembranous web which is found in the pharynx of diphtheria patients.)

The term **bacillus** derives from Latin *baculus*:"a small staff or rod" - and is virtually synonymous with the Greek *bakterion*. The genus *Spirillum* also comes from Latin: *spira* - "a coil" - as in the word **spiral**. The cocci originate from *kokkus*, which is Greek for "grain or kernel" - a name given to this unique organism in 1874 by **Theodore Billroth**, the father of modern abdominal surgery. (Billroth was a very close friend of **Johannes Brahms** - who frequently invited Billroth to appear as guest conductor for the Zurich Symphony Orchestra.)

The **Staphylococcus** descends from Greek - *staphyle*: "a bunch of grapes". The **Streptococcus** is obtained from the Greek *streptos*: "twisted, as in a necklace or chain". However the **gonococcus** exposes an error in medical lexicography. *Gone* is the Greek word for "seed" (e.g. **gonad**). Originally, it was mistakenly presumed that the urethral discharge in **gonorrhea** was due to the efflux of semen, rather than, as we now know, a mucopurulent inflammatory discharge. (*Rheos* is Greek for "flow", thus gonorrhea was a "flowing of seed, or semen". The **gonococcus** was therefore as mistakenly named as the disease that it causes.) *Rheos*, of course, may be found in countless words such as **leukorrhea** (*leukos*: Greek for "white"), **seborrhea** (*sebum* - Latin for "tallow or fat"), and **galactorrhea** (Greek *galaktos* : "milk". This also clarifies the word **galaxy**, which originally referred to our collection of local stars: the "Milky Way"). *Rheos* may also be found in **dysmenorrhea** (Greek *dys*: "abnormal,difficult,or painful" + *mensis* : Latin meaning "month"), **pyorrhea** (Greek *pyon* : "pus"), and **rhinorrhea** (Greek - *rhis* : "nose", as in **rhinoceros**. ("ceros" derives from Greek *keras*: "horny" - as in **keratin**, therefore, one might call this disagreeable animal a "horny nose"), and **logorrhea** (Greek *logos*: "word") i.e. a "diarrhea of words", something with which a constipation of ideas is occasionally associated.

Not only is the term **menses** directly from the Latin for month (sometimes referred to as "the monthlies"), but the word **moon** is as well. In fact, **month** derives from moon and refers to the period of one lunar cycle. One may find this relationship hidden within the expression "honeymoon". In early England it was customary for the newlyweds to share a glassful of mead or honey wine each night for the first month of marriage. Thus the harmony of their nuptials might be initiated and indelibly impressed on the marriage. In Italian it is called *luna di miele*: "month of sweetness".

It is, therefore, the "honey month". Or perhaps the honeymoonth.

The Electron and the X-ray

D.N.A. fragments are usually identified by the **Southern Blot** test. Restriction endonucleases are utilized to cut nucleoproteins into short segments. These segments are then separated by gel electrophoresis, and subsequently matched with R.N.A. target probes. This technique was first described by, and named for, British biologist **Edward M.Southern**. A comparable assay, which is used to identify proteins, has been lampooned "the Western Blot" test by some droll scientists from California.

The term **electrophoresis** derives from the Greek word *elektron*, which means "amber": the fossilized brownish resin often found along seacoasts. Now, the term **electron** refers to a negatively charged particle. This giant semantic leap in the connotation of "electron" stems from the fact that static electricity was originally discovered when **amber** was rubbed with a cloth. Thus, the electrical phenomenon shanghaied the native Athenian word, and forever altered its meaning.

The suffix of electrophoresis derives from the Greek *pherein*: "to carry". Therefore, electrophoresis means: "to carry a charge". (Christopher is "one who carries Christ". Semaphore is a "signal carrier" - from Greek *sema*: "sign". The field of **semantics** derives from the same root.)

Colloids are large molecules in suspension. When they are subjected to an electrical current, these molecules move toward the anode or the cathode side of the instrument, depending upon the net electrical charge on the surface of each particle. Arne Tiselius (1902-1971) first described and utilized electrophoresis in separating, identifying, and quantifying proteins, for which he was awarded a Nobel Prize in 1948.

The term **Colloid** may be traced to the Greek word *kolla*:"glue" + *oiedes*: "the same as, or like". Therefore, colloid means "glue-like", and refers to a thick, sticky mixture of insoluble particles.

Collagen, the fibrous protein substance within connective tissue, comes from *kolla: "glue"* + *gennao*: "to produce". Collagen, therefore means "to produce glue", and may be traced to the glutinous substance generated by boiling connective tissue, such as animal hides, a process perfected by Egyptians around 3000 B.C.

The root word *gennao* also occurs in **oxygen** and **hydrogen**. The Greek word *oxus*: "sharp" was used by **Antoine Lavoisier**, the "Father of modern chemistry", who mistakenly believed that oxygen was a constituent of all acids (this is actually true, instead, for hydrogen). *Oxus* - "sharp"- referred to the sour taste of all acids. (An **oxymoron** - such as "jumbo shrimp" - is a rhetorical expression containing contradictory terms. It is composed of Greek *oxus*: "sharp" + *moros*: "dull" (as in **moron**.) - that is, something both sharp and dull.) The term hydrogen is comprised of Greek *hydor*: "water" + *gennao*: "to produce", that is, "a substance which generates water".

Antoine Lavoisier, certainly one of the leading minds of his generation, was guillotined on May 8, 1794, during the "reign of terror", following the French Revolution. Joseph Lagrange, the eminent French astronomer, said of his contemporary Lavoisier: "A moment was all that was necessary to strike off his head, and probably a hundred years will not be sufficient to produce another like it."

A **collage** is created by gluing bits and pieces of art work together. The term *kolla* may also be detected by examining ancient Greek manuscripts. They often contained a page which was glued to the frontpiece, and which listed the contents of the manuscript. This page was called a *protokollon* from *proto*: "early or first" + *kolla* - that is, "first glued". Ultimately the English word **protocol** derives from this source. Colloid, collagen, collage, and protocol, therefore derive from a rather sticky common source.

In 1875,Sir William Crookes, an English physicist, (1832-1919) began a series of experiments using a glass tube, from which he had removed most of the air. He called this a **vacuum**_tube (Latin *vacuus*: "empty").One of his investigations led to the development of an ingenious toy known as a radiometer. (Tiny metal vanes colored white on one side and black on the other, spin around inside a vacuum glass cylinder when they are exposed to a light source.)

In a more important experiment, Crookes enclosed a **cathode** electrode within his vacuum tube. As he heated the electrode filament of this cathode, he observed a steady emission of electron radiation. Vacuum tubes such as these are called "Crookes' tubes". They have led to the development of incandescent light bulbs, oscilloscopes, and television receivers.

On November 5,1895, the chairman of the physics department at the University of Wurzberg, Germany entered a darkened room, and began a series of experiments using a Crookes' tube. He was particularly interested in luminescence, the induction of a glowing light from certain chemicals when they are struck by radiation from the cathode. On this particular day, the physicist had deliberately shielded his vacuum tube with black cardboard, in an attempt to block the transmission of electron radiation.

The cathode tube was turned on and a strange thing occurred. On the other side of the room, the target sheet of paper, coated with barium platinocyanide, began to glow brightly - despite the fact that the vacuum tube had been insulated with the black cardboard.

The German professor further discovered that a huge textbook interposed between the vacuum tube and the barium platinocyanide paper also failed to block the strange radiation that was being emitted. Most extraordinary of all was the physicist's observation that "if my hand is held before the fluorescent screen, the shadows show the bones darkly, with only faint outlines of the surrounding tissues."

Wilhelm Konrad **von Roentgen**, bewildered by the nature of this electromagnetic radiation he had accidentally discovered, called it an **x-ray**, because "X" had always signified an unknown quantity in mathematics. Roentgen composed only three papers on X-rays, but as a result of his work, became the first Nobel Laureate in Physics (1901). He donated all of his prize money to the University of Wurzberg.

Not long after Roentgen's seminal paper, Thomas Edison began experimenting with modified Crookes' tubes, using them as light bulbs and calling them "fluorescent lamps". However, he soon stopped the research. As he wrote: "I started in to make a number of these lamps, but I soon found that the x-ray had poisonously affected my assistant, Mr. Dally, so that his hair came out and his flesh commenced to ulcerate. I then concluded it would not do, and that it would not be a very popular kind of light, so I dropped it."

Mr. Dally died in 1904 at the age of 39, the first recorded fatality from man-made ionizing radiation.

One final note. The specific reason for which Sir William Crookes had developed his vacuum tube was to measure the mass of a newly discovered trace element. The vacuum tube would allow precise weighing of extremely small amounts of any substance, without the confounding buoyancy of air. Crookes had earlier discovered the new trace element in a sample of selenium ore. By spectroscopic analysis of the ore, he had observed a beautiful, thin, green line which did not correlate with any known substance. Crookes named the new element from the Greek word meaning "a green twig". He called it **Thallium**.

Cardiologists utilize a great deal of the stuff today. It may be the medical counterpart of the "greening of America".

The Numbers Game

A certain logic puzzle asks: "If the maximum number of hairs on a human head does not exceed 6,000,000, would it then be true that in the city of New York there must be at least two people with exactly the same number of hairs on his head?"

Numbers, digits, figures, tallies, amounts.

Our world is flooded with figures, deluged with digits, and nameless by the numbers.

But we are dysfunctional without them. From the sieve of Eratosthenes to quantum mechanics we depend on numbers to comprehend our universe - as well as to buy groceries.

Some 4000 years ago in the land between the Tigris and Euphrates rivers the Babylonian culture arose. (The area was known as **Mesopotamia** since it was *mesos* - Greek:"between" + *potomas* - Greek: "river", that is in the valley between two rivers. *Potomas* may be found hidden in the word **hippopotamus** - "river horse". Greek *hippos*: "horse" as in **hippodrome**, a place to run horses. Also, in the contraction *philo* - Greek: "to love" + *hippos*, which yields the name **Philip**: "one who loves horses").

One of the remarkable inventions of Babylonian culture was the **abacus**, a device that could perform sophisticated calculations. An abacus had parallel strings onto which were threaded colored pebbles. These could be moved rapidly along a row, each string representing numbers in the tens, hundreds, or thousands. **Calculation** and the **calculus** evolve directly from the abacus, a reference to those small stones on each string that were used for computation. (Latin - *calculus*: "a stone or pebble", which in turn derives from *calx*: "limestone", as in **calcium.**)

Digits are numbers, the term stemming from the ancient - and still popular - practice of counting on one's fingers. (Latin – *digitus*: "finger or toe".) A number consisting of two figures (e.g. 25) is a **binary** number. One of its two digits is known as a binary digit, the acronym for which is a **bit** in computer terminology. Eight bits constitute a **byte**, which is the basis for rating the memory capacity of a computer's hard disk (e.g. 200 megabytes - 200,000,000 bytes), or the size of a computer program (e.g. 700 kilobytes - 700,000 bytes).

Monos is the Greek word for "one". Its combining derivative is mono, as in **monocular**. **Monogamy** (Greek *gamos*: "marriage"), **monograph** (Greek *graphein*: "to write"), **monogram** (Greek *gramma*: "letter", as in **grammar** and **grammatical**), and **monologue** (Greek *legein*:"to speak") are also representative examples. A **monolith** is a figure made from a single stone, such as those at Stonehenge or Easter Island. (Greek *lithos*:"stone", as in the **Paleolithic** era, or in **nephrolithiasis** and **lithotripsy.**) A **monolithic** philosophy is unyielding and of a single dimension. **Mononucleosis** inundates the blood stream with white blood cells containing single nuclei (monocytes). A **monobactam**, such as Aztreonam, is a monocyclic beta-lactam.

The Latin for "one" is *unus*, as in the words **unilateral**, **universe**, and **uniform**. In our world there appear to be more mono's than uni's, but the choice keeps us from being too unidimensional or monotonous.

The prescriptive **Q.D.** stands for Latin *quaque die*:"every day", avoiding the need for either Greek or Latin numerals.

Duo is the Latin for "two", as in **duet**, **dual**, and **duplicate**. The **duodenum** was thought by early prosectors to have been twelve finger breadths long (Latin *duodeni* - "twelve", which in turn derives from *duo* + *decem*: "ten", that is, two plus ten). The prescriptive B.I.D. comes from the Latin *bis* ("twice") *in die*. The **Biceps** has two heads (Latin *bis* + *caput*:"head"),and a **bicuspid** valve or tooth possesses two points (Latin: *cuspis*). Severe aortic regurgitation causes the carotid pulse to become **bisferiens** (Latin *bis* + *ferio*:"to strike", that is the pulse is M-shaped, striking the finger twice during each systole).

A **biscuit** is something that is baked twice (Latin *bis* + *coctus*: "cooked or baked"). The Germans had a similar name for it - **zwieback**.

Tres is the Latin for "three", and yields the combining form **tri**. The **Triceps** has three heads, the **tricuspid** valve three cusps, and a **tripod** has three feet (Greek: *pous*: "foot"). A **Triangle** has three angles. **Trigonitis** is inflammation of the lower, triangular segment of the urinary bladder (*Tri* + *gonia* : "angle"). **Trigonometry** stems from *trigon* + *metron*: "measure", the measurement of three-angled structures. A **goniometer** is an orthopedic instrument which measures the angle, or range, of motion of a joint. **Nitroglycerine** is glyceryl **trinitrate**, which expands arteries or explodes buildings, depending on your specialty.

In ancient Rome, people often gathered on street corners to gossip and lament their circumstances - not unlike many of us today. In those days, three roads would often converge at a common intersection, which meant that early truants were able to loiter on three street corners at the same time (Latin - *trivium*: "place where three roads connect", which derives from *tri* + *via*: "road"). Thus the place at which those critical discussions were held, begot a word which best describes the speakers: **trivial**.

The Latin "four" is *quattuor*, in Greek it is *tettares*. The respective combining forms of each are **quadri** - and **tetra** -. A **quadrangle** is a plane geometric figure with four angles and four sides. A **quart** (Latin - *quartus*: "fourth")is one fourth of a gallon, and a **quartet** boasts four singers. A **quarter** horse is any breed of horse which reacts quickly to its rider's commands. These equines are used by both cowboys (and "city slickers") to herd cattle. The name arises from the horse's ability to accelerate quickly for up to a quarter of a mile.

Something which is said to be "**catty-cornered**" has four corners, from the French - *quatre*: "four", i.e. quatre-cornered. **Carillons** originally consisted of only four bells and were known by the Latin designation *quatternio*, which later evolved to the French carrignon, and finally to English carillon.

Quartan malaria (due to *Plasmodium malariae*) causes four day intervals of fever, the **quadriceps** is a four-headed muscle, and a **quadriplegic** has paralysis of all four extremities.(Greek - *plege*: "stroke". **Cycloplegia**, loss of visual accommodation, is due to paralysis of the ciliary muscle. *Cyclo* derives from the Greek *kyklos*: "circle", and refers in this case to the eye or ciliary muscle, which is round (as in **iridocyclitis**). The infamous **Ku Klux Klan** is also a derivative of *kyklos*, here referring to the inner circle of the Klan.)

The Greek word for "five" is *pente*, the combining form for which is **penta**. In Latin *quinque* is "five" and *quintus* means "fifth". In May 1934 a 24-year-old woman in Callender, Ontario delivered five babies: Emilie, Yvonne, Cecile, Marie, and Annette each averaging 2 pounds 11 ounces. The Dionnes became the world's first surviving **quintuplets.** (One hopes that the arrival of the McCaughey septuplets, in November 1997, has permanently eclipsed the old record.)

Ancient philosophers and alchemists believed that the universe was composed of four constituents - earth, air, fire, and water. However, they theorized that there must be a fifth element, the ultimate material from which the heavens were formed. They spoke of this fundamental substance as the *quinta essentia*: the fifth essence. It was, alas, never discovered but has given rise to **quintessence**, a word expressing the consummate manifestation or quality of a thing.

The **Pentagon** has five angles, as well as five sides. A **pentathlon** is an athletic competition with five events (*Greek* - *penta* + *athlon*: "prize or contest"). The **pentateuch** comprises the first five books of the Old Testament bible (Greek - *penta* + *teuchos*: "an implement or book"), known to the Jewish people as the Torah. **Pentobarbital** (Nembutal) is named for its five-carbon methylbutyl group which is attached to the parent barbituric acid nucleus. The intravenous anesthetic, **Pentothal**, is also named for its methylbutyl appendage, the "thal" resulting from **thio**barbiturate + the suffix "**al**". **Pentecost** is the fiftieth day after Passover, a Jewish holiday known as Shavuot. In the Christian religion, Pentecost is the seventh Sunday after Easter, consecrating the descent of the Holy Spirit upon the Apostles.

The Latin for "six" is *sex* as in **sextet**. A college **semester** comes from Latin *semestris*: "a six month or half-yearly period", which in turn results from Latin *sex* + *mensis*: "six months". (A **menstrual** cycle occurs monthly. The word *mensis* ultimately derives from the Greek word for "moon": *mene*.)

The *sexta hora* in ancient Rome was the sixth hour after sunrise. Since dawn was assumed to be 6:00 AM, the "sixth hour" was 12:00 PM. In southern climates the sun is almost directly overhead at noon, making energetic work difficult. That is how the **siesta**, the Spanish derivative of *sexta,* originated.

The word **noon** also has an interesting history. Originally the Latin term was *nona hora*: the "ninth hour" after sunrise, which would be 3:00 P.M. In the King James Bible, published in 1611, Mark's account of the crucifixion states: "there was darkness over the land until the ninth hour" (15:33). In the early Roman Catholic Church a daily service was conducted at that hour, and was called the **nones**, a contraction of *nona hora*. During the 12th century, however, this service was moved to an earlier hour. Eventually it was held at 12:00 P.M. thus that hour became the **nones**, or **noon**, hour.

The original Roman calendar had ten months and began with March. A Roman year looked like this :

March:	*Martius* : "of Mars".
April:	*Aprilis* : "second month".
May:	*Maia* the name of an earth goddess.
June:	For the goddess **Juno**, wife of Jupiter.
Quintilis:	Fifth month, later renamed for Julius Caesar and called **July**.

Sextilis: Sixth month, later renamed **August** for Augustus Caesar
September: *Septem* - "*s*even"
October: *octo* - "eight".
November: *novem* - "nine".
December: *decem* - "ten".

This last term became the basis for our **decimal** system, a **decibel**, a **decathlon,** and a **decade**. Boccaccio's **Decameron**, written in 1353, was a collection of tales narrated by a group of Italians during ten days of a plague epidemic. In ancient Rome, the victorious army arbitrarily executed every tenth prisoner, a policy known as **decimation**. Today it signifies virtual total annihilation.

The Roman year was only 304 days long, making it quite difficult for farmers who depend upon a solar year, to predict their planting season. In an unsuccessful attempt to rectify the problem, two additional months were added: **Januarius** and **Februarius**, named respectively for the two-faced god Janus, and Februa, the Roman festival of purification. Ultimately, January was assigned to begin each new year, since elected officials took office on the first of that month (even then the world seemed to revolve around politicians). Still the calendar did not operate properly, therefore, in 46 B.C. Julius Caesar ordered the astronomer Sosigenes to modify the calendar, in order to make it synchronous with the seasons. Sosigenes tried to accomplish the task by including 445 days in that year. The Romans called it the *year of confusion.*

Unfortunately, after all that work, the Julian calendar was still not coincident with the seasons. Thus, in 1582, Pope Gregory XIII formulated an entirely new calendar that did correct the problem. We continue to use it today, and call it the Gregorian calendar.

One may now appreciate why the names of our ninth, tenth, eleventh, and twelfth months are respectively derived from the numbers seven, eight, nine, and ten.

However, there is still that logic problem concerning the relationship between hairs on a head, and the population of New York City.

The answer, of course, is yes.

Shining Brightly

In ancient Rome one seeking elected office was required to wear a pure white toga to indicate his honesty and sincerity. Since he was arrayed in white he was called *candidatus* from the verb *candere*: "to shine", thus spawning the term **candidate**. Some might quarrel with the image in this case.

Several additional words emanate from *candere* - **candle**, and **incandescent** come quickly to mind. Indeed, Voltaire used rather satirical badinage when he entitled his parody of Leibniz' eccentric philosophy: "Candide". George Bernard Shaw did as much when dubbing his pungent burlesque of marriage: "Candida".

One wishes that our current politicians might at least exhibit as much **candor**. Humor may be too much to expect. (Perhaps they suffer from **candidiasis**!)

To be perfectly **candid**, however, the public did not treat Ex-Senator Joseph Biden very well after his gauche plagiary was uncovered. Other eminent politicians have been known to purloin a phrase or two from an eloquent predecessor. Consider, for instance, F.D.R. who is reverently remembered for - among other things - his haunting phrase : "We have nothing to fear but fear itself". Is it conceivable that Roosevelt might have snitched that remark from Henry Thoreau who, in an essay entitled "*A Week on the Concord and Merrimack Rivers*", had said : "Nothing is so much to be feared as fear." Or perhaps from an earlier work by the Frenchman Montaigne who, in 1590 wrote: "The thing of which I have most fear is fear".

Furthermore, consider a phrase from one of the greatest orators of this century, Winston Churchill, who spoke to England at the darkest hour of World War II. On May 13, 1940, in the House of Commons he said: "I have nothing to offer but blood, toil, tears, and sweat". Is it possible that Churchill might have borrowed that script - with slight modification - from Lord Byron's poem "*The Age of Bronze*". Here are the lines:

Safe in their barns, these Sabine tillers sent
Their brethren out to battle - Why? For rent!
Year after year they voted cent by cent,
Blood, sweat and tear-wrung millions - why? for rent!

They roared, they dined, they drank, they swore they meant
To die for England - why then live? - for rent!

Quite **candidly**, it appears that the most political rhetoric cannot be completely trusted to have its author's own metaphors, even in this "best of all possible worlds".

From Head to Foot

One of the unique signs of portal hypertension is the **caput medusae**, a cluster of dilated periumbilical venules. The name was obtained from its resemblance to Medusa, the mythological Gorgon, whose body was covered with dense scales, whose head was covered with snakes, and whose gaze turned people to stone. (The Gorgons were three hideous sisters, only one of which was mortal – Medusa. Her head was cut off by Perseus, according to Homer in The Iliad.)

The word *caput* in Latin means "head". Presumably the coiled, twisted, and distended abdominal vessels reminded some romantic clinician of Medusa's serpentine tresses.

Of course *caput* has spawned several words that we use more commonly. **Capitation** is a method of compensation by paying per head. Insurance companies have begun utilizing this method in an attempt to lower the costs of medical care. The headgear which men and boys wear for fun, a **cap**, also derives from *caput*. **Capital** punishment evolves from the rather nasty method of exterminating criminals - by **decapitation**. (Capital is also used to indicate the city that contains the head - although it's more often the seat - of government.) The leader of a military force, or of a large industry, is often called a **captain**.

Wealth in the form of money or property is also referred to as capital, since it belongs to one person. In Middle English the word evolved to **chattel**, referring to one's belongings or possessions. Thus the term chattel mortgage, to indicate a pledge of security based on moveable personal property rather than on real estate. In fact, a variant of chattel evolved into **cattle**, since these often represented a man's entire capital wealth. (The expression: **head of cattle**, therefore, becomes somewhat redundant.)

In the publishing industry, arranging an index by article headings was to **capitulate** them. Soon this word was employed to specify the terms of surrender - or "capitulation". When a French knight was outfitted from head to foot it was known as *cap - a - pie* (*pie* - from the Latin *pes*: "foot", which later became the French *pied.*) Cap - a - pie soon came to mean "in fine shape". But when Americans first heard the term they perceived it as "apple - pie". Thus the phrase – "**everything's in apple pie order**". Talk about murdering the king's English!

A bandage which is shaped like a cap and is used to cover a head wound, or the stump of an amputated limb, is called a **capeline**. (The material from which these bandages are often made is **gauze**, named for the middle eastern city from which it originated, **Gaza**, located in the renowned and troubled Gaza strip.) The Latin for bandage is *fascia*, a word which is also used to signify a sheet or bundle of fibers, as in **Buck's Fascia** of the penis. (Named for **Gurdon Buck**, a 19th century American surgeon.)

A cloak with a hood is called a **cape**. (See: Introduction) The word has evolved from Latin *caput* ("head", because of the accessory hood) through *cappa* to *capella,* and finally to the English term: cape. (A spit of land projecting into a body of water - a headland - is also known as a cape.)

"Pocks" – as in smallpox or chicken pox - stems from Old French *poque*, a pouch. (A *poquet* was a little pouch, or pocket.) The small pox was named to differentiate it from the "great pox" - Syphilis. (*Variola* was the Late Latin term for small pox, derived from *varius*: "spotted or varied". *Varicella* was the diminutive form of *variola.*) It was not until the ninth century that small pox was clearly described by the brilliant Persian physician **Rhazes**. And it was not until the late eighteenth century before William **Heberdon**, an English physician, differentiated chicken pox from small pox.

Heberdon, of course, is best remembered for his nine page paper entitled "*Some Account of a Disorder of the Breast*", read before the Royal College of Physicians in London, July 1768. This paper reported the first accurate clinical description of **angina pectoris** and ranks as an historic benchmark.

It may also be of some interest that following Heberdon's report Edward Jenner, a Gloucestershire practitioner, described the first thrombosed coronary artery in a man who had died of angina. Jenner, of course, is best remembered - not for contributions to early coronary pathology - but for his experimental use of Cow Pox (**Vaccinia**) in 1796 to immunize James Phipps against small pox. We seem to have come full circle.

The origin and development of words is often quixotic. The founder of Greek science, mathematics, and philosophy is said to have been the philosopher Thales of Miletus (624 B.C.-546 B.C.) Among his myriad accomplishments was the study of a black mineral obtained from Magnesia, a city in Asia Minor. Astonishingly, the substance was attracted to iron ore. Thales named it **magnes**. Today the mineral is known as **magnetite** and is the source of the word **magnet**.

Six hundred years later Pliny the Elder (23-79 A.D.) confused another black mineral substance with magnes and- adding to the confusion- misspelled its name, calling it **manganese**. It was finally correctly identified by Johan Gahn, a Swedish mineralogist, in 1774.

To further compound this rocky litany, a white rock had been discovered by the Romans during their occupancy of Magnesia. In 1831 a French chemist, Antoine Bussy, separated an element from this mineral. He named it **magnesium**. Today we use an oxide of magnesium (MgO) in suspension and call it **Milk of Magnesia**.

So from a rather unimportant ancient city in Asia Minor we have secured magnets, manganese, and magnesium - by hook and by crook and by serendipity.

And for constipation 30 ml. p.r.n.

The Magnificent Hoax

In ancient Greece, cosmologists believed that matter was composed of four fundamental elements: earth, air, fire and water. This left nothing to explain the nature of one's spiritual self, that God-searching, introspective philosopher within us all (exempting politicians).

Something else was clearly needed to satisfy that metaphysical requirement - the purest form of matter, fashioned from divine material. The cognoscenti selected **ether**, the imaginary material from which the heavens were thought to derive, as that substance. The Greeks called this divine substance *pempte ousia*. The Romans simply called it *quinta essentia*: the "fifth essence".And so they delivered to our modern world the **quintessence** of everything perfect.

Early physicians tried to explain illness in a similar manner. They envisioned the human as a receptacle containing four liquid substances (*humor*: Latin meaning "moisture or fluid") - each of which dictated a pattern of behavior. Balanced properly, the human remained well. However, an imbalance of these liquids led quickly to illness (one would be "out of humor"). There were four such humoral substances: blood, phlegm, yellow bile, and black bile.

An excess of blood would cause a person to be red-faced, warm, passionate, cheerful - in effect: **sanguine**.(Latin *sanguineus* - "blood"). A surplus of phlegm resulted in a taciturn, cold, aloof, reserved personality. In short one would be **phlegmatic.** An excess of yellow bile caused one to be bitter, sarcastic, hostile - in other words, to have a **bilious** personality and to assume a **jaundiced** view of the world. Lastly, a glut of black bile would result in depression, despair, and gloom. One would manifest **melancholy** (Greek *melanos*: "black" + *chole*: "bile".)

From the 16th through the 18th centuries, English comedies often relied heavily on such eccentric caricatures to goad audiences into roars of laughter - prompting critics to call these plays **humorous**.

Something, which cannot be called humorous, however, is the issue of scientific fraud. Unfortunately, within the past several years our profession has witnessed several disquieting instances of this behavior. One need only recall the recent case of a brilliant, young cardiologist, John Darsee, of Harvard Medical School, whose fabricated experiments resulted in his dismissal, followed by apologetic retractions from his distinguished superiors.

Yet scientific fraud has not been confined to the modern world. The greatest astronomer of ancient times - Claudius Ptolemy - did not make the planetary observations specified in his original data. He appears to have borrowed them entirely from the work of Hipparchus of Rhodes, an earlier astronomer. Instances of apparent deception have likewise been imputed to such scientific luminaries as Galileo Galilei, Gregor Mendel, John Dalton, and even an American Nobel Prize-winning physicist.

Perhaps the greatest scientific swindle of all time, however, took place at the beginning of this century. It involved a lawyer, an anthropologist, and a physician whose name may be familiar to you in quite a different context.

In 1856 workers discovered the skeletal remains of a human in the Feldhofer Cave, located seven miles east of Dusseldorf, Germany.The skull was smaller than average for an adult,and there were prominent supraorbital ridges and coarse cheek bones. Arguments mushroomed over the nature of this find. **Broca** believed the anatomy was that of an earlier species of man. **Virchow** disagreed. But it was finally established that the skeleton was an early specimen of *Homo Sapiens*.It was roughly 100,000 years old.

The cave itself was located near a stream in the Neander Valley therefore, the fossil was called **Neanderthal Man.** (German *thal*: "valley". The word is cognate with our term dale). In Czechoslovakia there is a valley named for St. Joseph (Joachims**thal**), which had become the location for a mint in the 16th century. A coin issued there was known as a **Joachimsthaler**, ultimately shortened to a **thaler**, and finally a **taler**. The Dutch called it a **daler** - and we refer to it as a **dollar**. Today one needs a valley full of them to buy anything.

Shortly after the discovery of *Homo Sapiens Neanderthalis* other skeletal finds were made in France, Italy, China, Africa and the island of Java. Marie Eugene Francois Thomas Dubois, a physician and lecturer in Anatomy at the University of Amsterdam, was impassioned over the idea that earlier forms of man (**Hominids**) might be discovered in caves, gravel beds, and rock strata - awaiting the probing eyes and hands of some fortunate paleontologist. He accordingly journeyed to the East Indies as a military surgeon. Once there he began his explorations on the island of Sumatra.

In 1890,on the island of Java, Dubois discovered a skull fragment, jaw bone and thigh. He believed them to represent the missing link between apes and hominids - the "ape-man" (*Pithecanthropus*: Greek *pithekos* - "ape" + *anthropos* - "man") - much better known to the world as the famous **Java Man**. Sometime later, in the Chou-k'ou-tien cave near Peking, China several additional skulls, mandibles and limbs were found which matched those of Java man. These quickly became designated **Peking Man**. Soon it became clear that none of these bones represented the postulated ape-man. Rather they were all remnants of an earlier hominid species, now known as *Homo erectus*.

We come then to the celebrated English hoax - perhaps the greatest scientific fraud ever committed. Near the end of the 19th century a rather obscure country solicitor lived and practiced law in County Sussex, England. He was a quiet and rather unpretentious man whose practice was quite modest and whose reputation quite unassuming.

However, he did enjoy one rather interesting diversion. He was an amateur geologist and anthropologist - a fossil hunter. In fact he had discovered the first Mesozoic animal in England, had reported it to the proper scientific societies and received appropriate commendation. The lawyer's name was **Charles Dawson**.

Dawson became friendly with a professional scientist - Arthur Smith Woodward - who headed the Department of Geology and Natural History at the British Museum. Dawson was profoundly convinced that specimens of primitive man would eventually be unearthed in England. (Until that time none had been found there, although monthly reports of such discoveries poured in from virtually every "uncivilized" country in the world.) Dawson tried to convince Woodward that England - that paradigm of intellectual excellence, the ground that spawned William Shakespeare and Isaac Newton - must ultimately prove to have been the nest of early man.

In 1898 Dawson became legal Steward of Barkham Manor, located in the small village of Piltdown. He discovered a large open gravel pit nearby - just the type that he believed might harbor the elusive skeletal finds he so desperately wished to locate.

In 1908 Dawson and a man named Samuel Allinson Woodhead, the local highschool chemistry teacher, began an intensive search of those gravel beds. Dawson was later joined by two Jesuit priests who were also nonprofessional, neophyte paleontologists.(One of them - **Father Pierre Teilhard de Chardin** - was to attain a measure of international stature for his theologic,philosophic,and paleontologic theories.He, in fact was one of those who discovered Peking Man.)

In July 1912 Dawson disclosed to Arthur Woodward that he had found a very primitive human skull and a mandible, which he believed might represent the Holy Grail of anthropologists - the missing ape-man link.

On December 18th 1912,at a meeting of the Geologic Society of London, this electrifying discovery was broadcast to the world. The bones were dark brown in color, mute testimony to their prehistoric age. Arthur Woodward and his associate Frank Barlow immediately began the task of reconstructing the face of this ancient ancestor, the common denominator between us and our nearest mammalian relatives.

Someone suggested that a professional anatomist might be useful in accomplishing this goal (Woodward was, after all, a geologist - not a biologist).It was quickly decided that the consummate choice would be the Conservator of the Hunterian Museum at the Royal College of Surgeons.

This gentleman was a physician graduate of the University of Aberdeen, previously chairman of the Department of Anatomy at London Hospital, and winner of the esteemed Strother's Prize for his elegant demonstration of the difference between the ligaments of men and apes. He had written extensively about the anatomy of the human heart with Sir James MacKenzie, and had studied with the famous anatomist Wilhelm **His** (of **Bundle of His** fame). In 1902 he had written the definitive text "*Human Embryology and Morphology*". In addition he had authored "*An Introduction to the Study of Anthropoid Apes*" (1897), "*Ancient Types of Man*" (1911),and "*The Antiquity of Man*"(1915). From 1914 - 1917 he was president of the Royal Anthropologic Institute, and for 23 years had been the editor of The Journal of Anatomy. For the *coup de Grace* he was a member of the Royal Society, president of the British Association for the Advancement of Science, and in 1921 received his Knighthood from King George V.

He was, in short, a reasonable choice to analyze the Dawson specimens and to determine their relationship to men and apes.

His conclusions were reached after exacting and meticulous reconstruction of the mahogany colored bones. The skullcap was clearly hominoid, the jaw with its worn down teeth, obviously ape-like. Yes, these skeletal fragments did indeed represent the long-pursued common ancestor of apes and men - "**the dawn man**".

They named it *Eoanthropus dawsoni*. (Greek *eos* - "dawn" + *anthropus* - "man"). The history of man had just been reshuffled. A new player had cast the die. And Charles Dawson beamed with satisfaction - it was the culmination of his dream.

Except.... except...for the doubts.Even from the beginning a few soft voices murmured uncertainly.Then,in 1924,Raymond Arthur **Dart**, a surgeon and anthropologist,discovered the famous **Taungs** skull that had been blasted out of limestone rock by miners in Africa,near a small village at the edge of the Kalahari Desert.He named it *Australopithecus africanus* (Latin **:** *austral* - "southern" + Greek :*pithekos* - "ape".The name **Taungs** comes from the name of the nearest railroad station serving the village.) Unexpectedly, Piltdown Man had become chronologically anomalous.

Stronger evidence emerged in 1953 when Kenneth Oakley.a geologist from the British Museum, analyzed the brownish pigment discoloring the Piltdown bones. It was found to be potassium dichromate - chemicals that had been deliberately used to stain the fossil bones in order to make them appear much older than they were.

The final confirmation of the stupendous deception was rendered in 1959. Carbon 14 dating proved that the ages of Piltdown's cranial vault and his jaw were millions of years apart. The jaw was authenticated as that of a fossil Orangutan.The skull was that of a modern man - possibly an Aborigine - that had been stolen years before from the British Museum.

Oh, yes. What about the celebrated anatomist, anthropologist, and physician who had declared Piltdown to be legitimate?

His name was **Arthur Keith** and with his student, **Martin Flack**, had been first to describe the Sino-Atrial Node of the human heart (Lancet 2:359,1906) - the **Node of Keith and Flack**.

Had Keith been a party to the magnificent deception? No one believes that. And besides, there was the presence of another mysterious and interesting figure - Sir Arthur Conan Doyle.

Doyle (b.May 22,1859,d.July 7,1930) had earned his doctorate in medicine at the University of Edinburgh. In 1891 he began an ophthalmology practice at Number 2 Devonshire Place - near Harley Street - in London, England. Unfortunately, his practice grew slowly. Therefore, he supplemented his meager income by writing detective stories. As his paradigm he used Joseph Bell, M.D., one of Doyle's finest and most astute medical professors, who was transmogrified into the great Sherlock Holmes of 221B Baker Street.

Sir Arthur's first novel was *A Study in Scarlet*, and it was a smashing triumph. Therefore, in 1890, flushed with financial success, Doyle retired from the practice of medicine to devote full time to fiction.

In addition to writing mysteries, Sir Arthur wrote science-fiction works such as *The Lost World* - which was ultimately made into a popular motion picture. He also authored historical works such as *Micah Clarke* and *The White Company* for which he fervently wished to be remembered - but which have long been virtually forgotten. In addition he wrote a number of pamphlets supporting England's decision to fight the Boer War, and he was an ardent spiritualist (particularly following his son's death in WW1).

Finally, and more to the present point, he fancied himself to be an amateur paleontologist.During the period of the Piltdown affair, Doyle was living in Crowborough,England, several short miles from the Piltdown quarries.He knew Dawson, and in fact had dined with him on several occasions.

In 1983, writing in the journal Science, two American archaeologists hypothesized that Arthur Conan Doyle may have actually masterminded this greatest of all scientific shams.(Winslow,J.H. & Meyer,A. "*The Perpetrator at Piltdown*" Science 4:32-43,1983)

But in 1990 Dr.Frank Spencer, Professor and Chairman of the Department of Anthropology at Queens College of New York, wrote a text entitled *Piltdown, a Scientific Forgery* (Oxford University Press), in which he shattered that hypothesis, stating quite clearly: ".....Doyle first learned of the (Piltdown) site's existence in the autumn of 1912, by which time Piltdown was an 'open secret'".

Whatever may be the actual truth, as with other great mysteries, this Magnificent Hoax will continue to captivate and tantalize - and to serve as the classic model of scientific fraud.

Eponyms II

"And if his name be George, I'll call him Peter
For new-made honor doth forget men's names"
Shakespeare

Eponyms, common nouns that once were proper names, are not always obvious. For example, in 1860 a German gynecologist described a method for compressing the post-partum uterus in order to discharge an obdurate placenta. The gynecologist was Karl Sigmund Franz Credé , and the procedure is identified with his name, although many physicians are quite unaware of its origin.

Another uncertain eponym, **Tourette's** Syndrome, is a rare neurological disease usually presenting in childhood with facial tics, grimaces, choreiform movements, echomimesia, echolalia, and coprolalia. George Edouard Albert Brutus **Gilles de la Tourette**, a neurologist at the famous Salpetriere Hospital in Paris, first described this bizarre illness in 1885. Some physicians have been unaware of its eponymic derivation.

(Incidentally, Tourette's hospital, the **Salpetriere**, had been originally built on the site of a former gunpowder storehouse, utilized by soldiers of Louis XIII. Salpetriere means "saltpeter", or potassium nitrate, an essential ingredient in gunpowder - the former gunpowder depot lending itself to the name of the hospital.)

Another uncertain eponym is the **Ghon** complex, a pulmonary lesion noted on chest xray, resulting from calcific deposits within an old granuloma. It was described in 1912 by Anton Ghon a Professor of Pathology at Prague University. (Ironically, Ghon died of tuberculous pericarditis in 1936.)

A **Pancoast** tumor is characterized by shoulder and arm pain in the distribution of the ulnar nerve, a **Horner's Syndrome**, and a carcinoma within the superior sulcus of the lung. It was described by Dr. **Henry K.Pancoast**, who was the first physician in the United States to be appointed as a professor of radiology. (University of Pennsylvania.)

(**Horner** was a Swiss ophthalmologist who first described the ptosis, enophthalmos, and meiosis caused by a lesion of the cervical sympathetic nerves.)

Dr. **Ernest Goodpasture** first described the syndrome of intrapulmonary hemorrhage, hemoptysis, and glomerulonephritis. He graduated Johns Hopkins University, and for 30 years was professor of pathology at Vanderbilt University. Nonetheless, the eponymic origin of the **Goodpasture Syndrome** often passes unrecognized.

In ischemic heart disease, a classic ECG abnormality consists of upward bowing of the ST-T segment with inversion of the T wave. This is known as the **Pardee Sign**, after Harold Ensign Bennett **Pardee**, a Manhattan cardiologist who described it in 1920.

(During World War I, Pardee collaborated with Sir Thomas Lewis in delineating the "soldier's heart syndrome", also known as neurocirculatory asthenia. This condition had originally been described in Civil War soldiers by Jacob Mendes **Da Costa**, and is often referred to as **Da Costa's Syndrome**. Today it may maquerade as chronic fatigue.)

Eponyms may originate from the names of places as well as people. The *Coxsackie* virus represents an assorted group of enteroviruses that are named for **Coxsackie**, New York, a small town on the Hudson River that lies just north of Catskill, N.Y. The virus was originally recovered from a patient who lived there.

(Enteroviruses are those which reside primarily in the intestines. From Greek: *enteron*: "intestine". Enteroviruses are a subgroup of **picornaviruses,** which also include the poliovirus and echovirus families. Picornavirus derives from Spanish *pico*: "small" (as in a picosecond which is one trillionth or 10^{-12} seconds) plus RNA, since the virus contains ribonucleic acid. Thus a picornavirus is a very small, RNA-containing virus. The poliovirus is named for the disease which it causes. **Poliomyelitis** is derived from Greek *polios:* "gray",and *myelos*: "marrow", referring to the gray matter of the central nervous system which is infected by the virus. Ancient physicians believed that the brain and spinal cord were the "marrow" contained within the skull and vertebral column. The root *myelo-* also refers to the bone's marrow, as in **myelocyte, myeloma, myelofibrosis**, etc.

(The **echovirus** is an acronym for enterocytopathic human orphan + virus. The "orphan" status was specified because no human disease had been associated with the virus when it was initially discovered.)

Epidemic pleurodynia, caused by a *Coxsackie* B virus, should be suspected in patients with fever and pleuritic chest pain. The viral agent responsible was initially recovered from patients who inhabited Bornholm, a small Danish island in the Baltic Sea. Therefore, the eponymic **Bornholm's** Disease.

The diminutive deer tick, *Ixodes dammini*, will occasionally infect its human host with the spirochete *Borrelia burgdorferi*. The resulting illness frequently begins with a classic rash (erythema chronicum migrans) followed by severe arthritis, associated with occasional meningitis, and myocarditis. The disease was first identified within a cluster of school children living in Lyme, Connecticut. Thus the eponym **Lyme Disease**.

Perhaps the greatest source of unrecognized eponyms might be found in the taxonomy of microorganisms. For example, Amadee **Borrel**, a French bacteriologist, for whom the genus *Borrelia* was named, and Daniel **Salmon**, an American veterinarian, for whom the genus *Salmonella* was designated. So, also, were *Escherichia, Brucella, Giardia, Klebsiella, Neisseria, Shigella, Nocardia, Wuchereria, Bordetella, Bartonella, and Listeria* derived. They emerged from such progenitors as:

Theodor **Escherich**, a distinguished German pediatrician who discovered *Escherichia coli* in 1886, and Major-General Sir David **Bruce** who discovered the bacterium responsible for Undulant Fever, while stationed on the island of Malta. The disease was also called Malta Fever. (In cattle it is known as **Bang's Disease**, named after a Danish veterinarian, Bernhard Lauritz **Bang**.) The disease is also called Brucellosis. Years later, while stationed in Zululand, Bruce discovered that the tsetse fly carried African sleeping sickness. *Trypanosoma brucei rhodesiense* and *gambiense* are the infectious organisms.

Alfred Mathieu **Giard** was a famous 19th century French biologist.(The species name for *Giardia lamblia* emanates from William **Lambl**, an Austrian physician who first distinguished the causative agent in a patient with Giardiasis.)

Theodor Albrecht Edwin **Klebs** was a German bacteriologist who discovered the Diphtheria organism (It is also known as the **Klebs-Loeffler bacillus**. Friederich **Loeffler** was another German bacteriologist who first cultured the diphtheria organism. He should not be confused with the Swiss physician who described an eosinophilic pneumonia - William Loeffler).

Albert Ludwig Sigesmund **Neisser** - German dermatologist who discovered the gonococcus.

Kiyoshi **Shiga** - Japanese bacteriologist who first described a bacillus which causes dysentery. In 1919 it was named for him.

Edmond **Nocard** - French veterinarian who first isolated the fungous that now bears his name.

Otto **Wucherer** - German physician who discovered the filarial parasite that causes elephantiasis.(The species name of *Wuchereria* *bancrofti* derives from Joseph **Bancroft** , a British physician who had independently discovered the filarial organism.)

Jules Jean-Baptiste-Vincent **Bordet** - Belgium bacteriologist and immunologist, discovered (together with Octave **Gengou**, a French bacteriologist) the organism responsible for whooping cough - the bacillus - now named *Bordetella pertussis*. In 1919 Bordet received the Nobel Prize in Medicine.

Alberto **Barton** - Peruvian physician discovered *Bartonella bacilliformis*, the organism that causes **Oroyo Fever**.

Joseph **Lister** - British surgeon who introduced aseptic surgery to the world.

And the list goes on. Eponyms unrecognized. Faceless names, no longer remembered.

Like bloomers, bikinis, and jerseys, people will continue to endow prosaic objects with proper names - subsidizing common idiom with quite uncommon sources.

Turning Points

We inhabit a whirling globe that is somewhat askew. Careful measurement of earth's north-south axis relative to the sun's polar axis, confirms this tilt. At its maximum, earth inclines some 23.5 degrees from our aging star.

In summer the northern half of earth slopes toward the sun. In winter it leans away. At noon on June 21st of every year - the first day of summer - the sun hovers directly above the latitude 23.5 degrees north of the equator. (23.5 degrees north latitude is known as the Tropic of Cancer.) Conversely, at noon on December 22 - the first day of winter - the sun is directly above the Tropic of Capricorn, 23.5 degrees south latitude.

The sun reaches its lowest point in the sky on that first winter day. Thereafter, it begins to rise higher and higher above the horizon. Upon reaching its summer zenith the sun begins a slow daily descent, once again touching its nadir on December 22nd.

This annual ritual is repeated inexorably. And a curious phenomenon occurs as the sun reaches the limit of each excursion in winter or summer - it appears to pause at that position for a few days before starting to backtrack. This apparent hesitation in the sun's bounce is known as the summer or winter **solstice.** (From the Latin *sol* : "the sun" and *sistere*: "to pause or stand". For just a day or two, the sun appears to **stand still** above the horizon. Armistice has the same terminal root meaning "a pause or stoppage of arms" - an archaic term we seem to have little use for today.)

The latitude at which either summer or winter solstice occurs is known as a **tropic** - the place where the sun appears to turn in the sky. (Greek: *tropos*: "a turning" - e.g. phototropic: "turning of plants toward the light", heliotropic: "turning toward the sun". One may also include corticotropin, gonadotropin, thyrotropin, and somatotropin - each of which "turns" a target gland toward production of a certain hormone.). The zone between these two earthly "turning" latitudes (the tropic of Cancer and Capricorn) is therefore known as "the tropics".

At noon on the first day of fall or spring (September 23rd and March 21st respectively) one will find the sun directly above the equator.

This day is known as the autumnal or vernal **equinox**, and both daytime and nighttime are 12 hours long.(Latin: *aequus*:"equal" + *nox*:"night").

Ancient astronomers carefully studied the motion of the sun, moon, and five visible planets. They also examined collections of distant stars which they called **constellations** (Latin *con*: "together" + *stella*: "stars"),often imagining them to be animals, such as Ursa Major (the bear),Taurus (the bull),Leo (the lion),and Cancer (the crab).

The word **cancer** was first used by Galen to indicate a malignancy. He described a breast tumor thus: "As a crab's feet extend from every part of the body, so in this disease the veins are distended, forming a similar figure." The hardness of the tumor furthered the simile by suggesting a crab's shell.(The Greek word for crab is *karkinos* which created the term **carcinoma.)**

Painful, indurated oral ulcerations - although non-malignant - were also named for the crab. They were called **cankers.** In addition, the French termed the hardened, primary lesion of syphilis a **chancre** in resemblance to those seashore arthropods. Thus cancer, canker, and chancre are all rooted in the same crustacean metaphor.

Early astronomers had also noted that every **eclipse** of the sun or moon occurred within a very narrow segment of the sky. This slender zone was referred to as the **ecliptic**, and it corresponds to the annual path of our bouncing ball of fire as it meanders through the heavens. (Eclipse is from Greek *ek*: "out" + *leipein*: "to leave",that is, during an eclipse the moon or sun appears to have been left out of the sky.)

Within the ecliptic pathway, twelve constellations were found and named - one for each month of the year. Most of these constellations were designated for animals. The entire collection of twelve constellation was called the **zodiac** (Greek *zodion* from *zoion*: "animal" - as in **zoology** - plus *kuklos*: "circle". Hence the zodiac is "a circle of animals").

Returning briefly to the root word *tropos*, Greek mythology speaks of **Atropos** - one of the Three Fates - who, with her macabre sisters Clotho and Lachesis, were believed to control the destiny of every human. Clotho held a spindle and onto it she could spin the thread of life. Lachesis would measure and determine its ultimate length. But it was Atropos who cut the thread. There was then no turning back.(Greek *a*: "not" + *tropos*: "turning")

Atropine ($C_{17}H_{23}NO_3$), an alkaloid found in *Atropa belladonna*, is a member of the deadly Nightshade family. It is named for the venomous sister Atropos. Administered in sufficient dose it too will cut the thread of life.

The Nightshades are plants within the order *Solanaceae*. This order embraces prominent dietary staples including the Irish potato, the red pepper, and the tomato. Included as well are the tobacco plant and the **Jimson** weed. This last plant, *Datura stramonium*, is occasionally responsible for poisoning small children and animals. Jimson was initially discovered around Jamestown, Virginia, and was known as Jamestown weed. Through the years its name has become shortened to the colloquial "Jimson" weed. Its leaves, flowers, and seeds contain up to 0.45% belladonna alkaloids, mostly atropine, hyoscyamine, and scopolamine. **Locoweed** - from the Spanish *loco*: "crazy" - another deadly plant that is in the pea family, contains mainly scopolamine.

The toxicity of belladonna plants has been known for centuries. From the era of the Roman Empire and through the Middle Ages, these plants were often used for political assassination. (Hamlet's father was said to have been poisoned by a mixture of **Henbane** poured into his ear by his brother Claudius. If you have doubts about the possibility of this method of envenomation, think about what might occur in the event of a ruptured tympanic membrane, and a patent Eustachian tube.)

Henbane is officially *Hyoscyamus niger,* and is a chief source of the belladonna alkaloid **hyoscyamine**. (Greek - *hyoskyamos*: "pig bean", a reference to its obnoxious odor.) The name henbane alludes to the effect of its poison on chickens. **Bane** is old English, meaning, deadly poison, the cause of death, or ruin, as in "it's the bane of my existence." Dogbane has a similar implication.

Belladonna alkaloids act as anticholinergics and antimuscarinics. **Cholinergic** refers to the neurotransmitter acetylcholine. **Muscarine** is an alkaloid, first derived from the toxic mushroom *Amanita muscaria* by Schmiedeberg in 1869. *Muscaria* is Latin for "pertaining to flies". Extracts of the mushroom had been used for centuries as a natural pesticide, known to kill flies. (Latin *musca*: "fly". In Spanish, the term is *mosca,* from which we derive the diminutive term **mosquito**: "little fly".)

Acetylcholine is the neurotransmitter released by both pre- and post-ganglionic fibers of the parasympathetic nervous system. Muscarine duplicates the effect of such stimulation, while atropine inhibits those muscarinic effects. (The nicotinic action of acetylcholine on the somatic motor terminals is not blocked by atropine at usual therapeutic doses.)

The parasympathetic nervous system includes neural outflow from the mid-brain via the nucleus of Edinger-Westphal and the Oculomotor Nerve. (Ludwig **Edinger** 1833-1918, was a German neurologist who founded comparative neuro-anatomy. Karl Friedrich Otto **Westphal**,

1833-1890, was the first professor of neurology appointed in Berlin. He described the nucleus in adults two years after Edinger had initially described it in a fetus.)

The parasympathetic system also includes elements of the 7th cranial nerve (Chorda tympani), and the 9th,and 10th (Vagus) nerves. (**Vagus** - Latin meaning "wandering", a reference to the meandering, lengthy course of the nerve. Someone who is **vague** also meanders in a discursive, rambling fashion.)

Within the intestine, the Vagus fibers innervate Auerbach's and Meissner's plexus, releasing acetylcholine from post-ganglionic terminals. (Leopold **Auerbach**,1828-1897, was a professor of neuropathology in Breslau, Germany. Georg **Meissner**,1829-1905,was professor of anatomy and physiology at Basle and Gottingen. In addition to describing the submucous plexus in the gut, he also described the touch nerve endings in the skin, called Meissner's Corpuscles.)

The parasympathetic system ends with sacral nerves II - IV, innervating bladder, rectum and sexual organs.

Atropine blocks the cholinergic and muscarinic effects of this system, resulting in several consequences. As the dose reaches increasingly toxic levels, there is progressively: sinus tachycardia, dryness of the mouth, mydriasis,blurring of vision,difficulty in swallowing,hot and dry skin, ataxia, restlessness, hallucinations, delirium, coma, respiratory arrest and death.

Classic atropine toxicity may be described as: "hot as a hare", "blind as a bat", "dry as a bone" , "red as a beet", and "mad as a wet hen!"

Scopolamine derives from plants of the genus *Scopolia,* named for the Italian Botanist G.A.**Scopoli.**

Belladonna (Italian: "beautiful lady") is named for its early use as a cosmetic, which results in beautiful eyes with very large, dilated pupils.

These, too, have occasionally been known to be turning points.

The **tragus** is the small cartilaginous projection anterior to the external meatus of the ear. It is often covered with **tragi**, which are small hairs growing over the surface of the pinnae.

(*Pinna* - Latin for "feather" The pinnae of the ears are sort of "wings" that project from our head., and since a bird's wing is largely comprised of feathers, the analogy was carried to completion by the presence of these tiny hairs. The word **pen** derives directly from *pinna*, and originally referred to the feathered or quill pen.) Tragus developed from the Greek word *tragos*: "goat". An imaginative, early prosector must have visualized a goat's chin and beard as he described the external ear. A **tragedy** is literally "a goat's song" deriving as it does from Greek *tragos* + *oide* ("song"). It has its origin in the ancient Greek chorus, whose dramatic function was to mock fate. These plays often dealt with great misfortune and sorrow, and the chorus members frequently portrayed satyrs, dressing themselves in goatskins for the part. The term *tragos oides* ultimately was applied to the entire play (*Oide* – "song" is found in the term **ode**, as in those written to a Grecian urn, or a Nightingale.)

The Greek god of forests and wild animals was **Pan.** He was the patron of shepherds and hunters and flaunted the ears, horns, tail and inguinal parts of a goat. The less spectacular aspects of his anatomy were those of a man. He was playful, frisky, lustful, libidinous, and unpredictable. One of his favorite diversions was to frighten unwary travelers as they wandered through his forest. Hence he incited **panic**.

Pan was one of a group of woodland deities known as **satyrs**. They attended **Bacchus**, god of wine,(the "**Bacchanalia**" was a Roman festival - an orgy of drinking and eating). Pan and his friends are famous for a disorder known as **satyriasis**, which requires a goat-like constitution as well. It is the masculine counterpart of **nymphomania**. The Romans also venerated Pan, but they renamed him **Faunus**. Debussy's orchestral work *Prelude a l'apres-midi d'un faune* (Prelude to Afternoon of a Faun) exalted these woodland creatures.

In addition, the renowned Swedish physician and botanist, Dr. Carl Von Linne, immortalized these woodland deities in his seminal classification of plants and animals calling them flora and **fauna**.

(Incidentally, you may know Von Linne only by his latinized name, a convention of his era. It is **Carolus Linnaeus.**)

A number of geographic names stem from mythology. **Phoenix** (Arizona), for instance, is named for an ancient Egyptian bird that built its own funeral pyre, died, and arose from its own ashes. Europe derives from **Europa**, a Phoenician princess who was kidnaped by Zeus. **Olympia** (Washington) stems from **Mount Olympus**. **Rome** was built by **Romulus** and named after its mythical creator.

Medicine has a lexicon of words that have descended from early mythology. **Asklepios**, the legendary Greek physician (also called Aesculapius), was the son of Apollo, and also the Greek god of Medicine. He was taught the art of healing by Chiron the Centaur, who had also tutored Hercules, Aeneas (of Virgil's "Aeniad"), and Achilles. Asklepios is most often depicted in a flowing white robe, holding a cane that has a single snake coiled around it.

A winged staff with two serpents entwined about it, on the other hand, was the famous **Caduceus** of **Mercury**, who was the messenger of the gods. (He was also known as **Hermes**, to the Greeks).

Originally, the staff of Asklepios was the official seal of the U.S. Surgeon General's office, and the universal symbol for medicine. However, in 1871, the Surgeon General mistakenly replaced the single serpent with dual reptiles intertwined on a winged staff, which represents the Caduceus of Hermes. This change was done for aesthetic reasons, and would ordinarily not be terribly disconcerting, unless you remember that Mercury was the god of trade, of commerce, and of wealth. He was, unfortunately, also the god of thieves. His duties, moreover, included placing his serpentine wand over the eyes of the newly deceased, and escorting them into Hades!

One suspects that this distinguished medical symbol could have been chosen more carefully.

Asklepios, as mythology relates, was physician to Jason and his Argonauts. If you recall, these adventurous sailors undertook a dangerous journey to obtain the Golden Fleece - the coat of a ram that had safely flown two young people - Phrixus and his sister Helle - away from their murderous uncle.(**Helle**, unfortunately, fell into the sea and drowned, which resulted in the naming of that body of water the **Hellespont** – Greek for "Helen's Sea".) The Argonauts discovered the golden fleece in **Colchis**, a region at the eastern end of the Black Sea, now part of the Republic of Georgia, and formerly part of the U.S.S.R.

A lovely flower grows in that part of the world. It is a member of the lily family, blooms in late autumn, and brandishes an array of pink, purple, and white petals. The plant is named for the region: *Colchicum autumnale*. One of its primordial secrets lies in its underground root, which, when eaten, exhibits anti-inflammatory properties. Asklepios often used it to treat rheumatism and gout. In 1763,von Storck promoted this chemical for the treatment of gout, calling it *colchicum*. Ben Franklin used it himself, and introduced it into the United States. In 1820 it was purified, and the drug produced was named **colchicine**. .Early physicians believed that gout was caused by specific humors (liquids), which trickle out of the body, drop by drop. The Latin for "drop" is *gutta*, from which **gout** ultimately evololved.. Gutta also gave us "**gtts**" (drops) as a prescriptive term.

Colchis was located south of the Caucasus Mountains. It was in those Caucasus Mountains that Zeus had chained Prometheus for giving man fire. And it was also in those craggy peaks that a human skull was once discovered.

The skull was prehistoric but quite well preserved, and it was sent to a scientist for careful study. His name was Johann Friedrich Blumenbach, and he is considered the father of physical anthropology. He was the first man to suggest that humans might be evaluated through comparative anatomy. And he was first to classify human subspecies (or "races") by anthropometric measurements of their skulls.

Based on those measurements, he suggested that there were five families of man: brown (Malaysians), red (American Indians), yellow (Mongols), black (Ethiopians), and white. The last he named Caucasian, because the most perfect example of its skull had come from the Caucasus Mountains.

Unfortunately, although Blumenbach did not intend it, his theory has subsidized centuries of bigots who have used it to advance the dogma of racial inferiority - from the ignominy of American slavery - to the perfidy of the Holocaust. He also inadvertently provided physicians with their most consecrated pomposity - heard at almost every case presentation - "A well-developed, well-nourished Caucasian....". And lest we not forget, the tedious drone of the police dispatcher who also uses the same cliche/: "Male Caucasian, five foot eight,165 pounds...."

Asklepios had two daughters **Hygeia** and **Panacea** who are known to physicians and their patients alike, and who have given us two excellent eponymic nouns.

Mercury (Hermes), in addition to his courier position, was also the father of Greek alchemy. Alchemists were sorcerers, pseudoscientists, and magicians, but were nonetheless the first craftsmen to soften metals by utilizing an intense heat source. And they learned how to use the hot molten ore to fasten objects tightly together - such as the lid on a jar. This process has become known as **hermetic** sealing.

Aphrodite, one of the twelve Olympic gods, was famous for her beauty and her promiscuity. She had reluctantly married the grotesque and repulsive **Vulcan**, god of fire (**volcano** and **vulcanism**), hence she found need to import comely paramours to gratify her carnal desires. Occasionally she resorted to **aphrodisiacs** in order to achieve these ends.

Among her lovers was Hermes with whom she conceived a son. The baby was named for both parents - **Hermaphroditus**. As he grew into handsome maturity, Salmacis, a water nymph, fell in love with him but could not tolerate a moment's separation from her sweetheart. She, therefore, merged her spirit with his. Salmacis and her lover thus occupied the same body, which developed both male and female sexual characteristics - a **hermaphrodite**.

Aphrodite was known as **Venus** to early Romans.. She was the goddess of beauty, the mother of love, and the mistress of pleasures. One of her children was **Eros**, the god of love. A second child was **Hymen**, the god of marriage. The third child was **Priapus** - god of fertility. **Priapism, hymen**, and **erotic** are their medical cognates. In addition, Venus gave us a wealth of **venereal** diseases as well.

Other characters from ancient mythology have augmented our medical vocabulary, such as **Psyche**, goddess of the human soul, and **Narcissus**, a beautiful youth who fell in love with his own reflection. One must also include the sea god **Proteus**, who had the ability to assume various shapes. The bacterial genus *Proteus* was named for him. And we can credit him also with that ubiquitous expression of sophomoric rhetoric, often heard at grand rounds: "the protean manifestations of disease".

Saturn was the Roman god of agriculture. His temple served as the Roman state treasury, and its vestiges may still be found at the west end of the Forum. A great festival, the Saturnalia, was held each December in his honor. It was the most popular and joyful of Roman festivals. Commerce was suspended, slaves were granted temporary freedom, moral constraints were relaxed, and gifts exchanged.

During that era, astronomers became aware of five unique celestial objects. They already knew that stars were "fixed" in their position, each relative to the others, and that they rotated nightly from east to west in the dome of the sky. This was true for most stars, but not for five idiosyncratic "stars" that appeared to wander aimlessly through the heavens, pursuing their own enigmatic destinies. The primitive stargazers called these bizarre objects **planets** (Originally these were called *astroplanetes*, Greek - *Astron*: "star"+ *planetes*: "wanderers".) One of these - the outermost planet visible to the naked eye - was named Saturn, in honor of their god. It was a very slowly moving celestial body, hence the alchemists hypothesized that it must be made of lead, which was the heaviest known element of that era. Therefore, to have a **saturnine** disposition meant to have a plodding, morose, and rather gloomy personality.

In addition, chronic lead poisoning became known as **saturnism** and (since we now realize that lead hinders the excretion of uric acid) the resulting illness is called **saturnine gout**.

Of course, the definitive Latin word for lead is *plumbum,* from which our chemical symbol **Pb** is derived. This explains the alternate term for lead toxicity - **plumbism**. It also explains why one calls a **plumber** when the pipes leak - since all water pipes were originally fabricated from lead. (Someone has even suggested that this might explain the fall of the Roman Empire.)

Finally, you may suspect why that lovely home you have just built exhibits such a paucity of true right angles. The builder obviously had failed to hang a heavy lead weight onto a string, in order to obtain a perpendicular. He had not used a **plumb line.**

The Romans thought so much of Saturn that they named one day of their week after him: *dies Saturni*. This ultimately became **Saeturndaeg** in Old English and, finally Saturday. Sunday was originally the "sun's day", Monday the "moon's day". The other four days of the week were named respectively for Mars (*dies Martis;* in French it became *Mardi*, thus Mardi gras or *Mardi gros* – "fat Tuesday" – which initiates the Christian season of Lent), Mercury, Jupiter, and Venus. Ultimately, five Roman days were replaced by their Anglo-Saxon (Teutonic) cognates: *Tiu* the Norse god of war (*Tiu's daeg* or Tuesday), *Wodin* the king of all the Norse gods (*Wodin's daeg* or Wednesday), *Thor* the Norse god of thunder (*Thor's daeg* or Thursday), and *Frigga*, Wodin's wife and goddess of love (*Frigga's daeg* or Friday). Remember these derivations next time you expound on our Western scientific and cultural "sophistication".

Returning for a moment to goats, Zeus, the chief god of the Greek pantheon, possessed a magnificent shield that protected him from any harm. The shield – known as *aigis* - was forged out of the hide of a goat named **Amalthea**, who had suckled Zeus as an infant. All who were under that shield were symbolically under divine protection. The term: "**aegis**" derives from that mythology.

Booze, Bloodshed and Bounty

Since the Middle Ages it has been customary for a noble patrician to give his wife a gift on the morning after their wedding. In Germany this was known as a *morgangabe* - "a morning gift" If the bride were a commoner, or from royalty far below her husband's status, that auroral gift was all she could expect from her aristocratic spouse. Neither she - nor any of their offspring -would ever acquire his rank or share in the royal legacy.

In Latin such an alliance was known as *matrimonium ad morganaticum* - "marriage based on the morning gift." Today it is simply known as a **morganatic** marriage.

As if to emphasize the inequality between them, during the ceremony the groom would offer his left hand to the bride. Such rituals were contemptuously called "left-handed marriages," which ultimately spawned the expression: "**a left-handed compliment**" - an insult cloaked in thinly veiled flattery.

In the early years of the 20th century, a morganatic marriage took place between Archduke Francis Ferdinand, heir to the Austro-Hungarian throne, and Sophie Chotek, a déclassé countess. Their wedding would have been but a trivial footnote to European history, and of absolutely no consequence to the rest of the world, were it not for two terrifying minutes on the afternoon of June 28, 1914.

During the preceding eighteen months, the Balkan League, which was comprised of Serbia, Bulgaria, Albania, and Greece, had defeated the Turkish Ottoman Empire. Following that triumph, however, the victors began to quarrel among themselves.

A savage Balkan war burst forth. Reports of atrocities between Bulgarians and Serbs were commonplace. The Russians, who had intimate connections to the Serbians, attempted unsuccessfully to mediate. The Austro-Hungarians, always the opportunists, were busily annexing unprotected Balkan territory.

Finally, Great Britain negotiated an armistice agreement, but it was an uneasy truce, and - at that fragile political moment - Archduke Ferdinand and his wife decided to pay a state visit to Sarajevo.

Their parade route led directly past a cafe called Zeata Moruna, the "Green Garland." Inside the cafe, sipping coffee was a nineteen-year-old

Serbian highschool student named Gavrilo Princip. Several weeks before, Princip and his friends had been ushered into a concealed, dimly lit room. There, lying on a small oak table, were a skull, a gun, a bomb, and a vial of cyanide poison. And there, in that secret chamber, they had sworn the Oath of the Black Hand. The Black Hand was a brutal terrorist organization led by a Colonel Dragutin Dimitrijevic, and the oath went as follows:

> "By the sun which warms me, by the earth which feeds me,
> by God, by the blood of my ancestors, by my honor, and by
> my life, I swear fidelity to the cause of Serbian
> nationalism, and to sacrifice my life for it."

The Archduke and his wife were sitting in an open "Graf und Stift" automobile. Princip calmly approached the vehicle and fired seven shots at the occupants. The Archduke was hit in the neck and died almost instantly. His wife Sophie, shot in the abdomen, died on the way to a hospital.

One month later Austria-Hungary declared war on Serbia, Russia invaded Germany, and Germany declared war on Russia and France. World War One had started.

Four years later 20 million people were dead.

80 years later - *deja vu.*

War, of course, is a state to which no one admits allegiance. Yet it seems to be an essential human nutrient, for we appear incapable of an enduring existence without it.

Count some of the wars we list among our cherished historic possessions:

The Babylonian War
The Hittite War
The Trojan War
The Messinian War
The Ionian War
The Peloponnesian War
The Punic Wars
War of Roses
Spanish-American
Napoleanic
French and Indian
American Revolutionary

The Arab-Israeli, Iran-Iraq, Italo-Ethiopian, Korean, Vietnam, Persian Gulf, World Wars I and II. And let's not forget the 7-Year, 30-Year, and 100-Year Wars. Nor should we slight the various civil wars such as the English, Chinese, Spanish, Mexican, Russian, French, Rhodesian, and the American Civil War. This, by the way, is only a partial list of the slaughter, bloodshed, and carnage - following which each participating nation thoughtfully builds such handsome and poignant memorials.

I have not included the more trivial military campaigns that have inspired patriots and mesmerized throngs of faithful posterity.

For example, there was the curious incident that had occurred on board the British ship **Rebecca** in 1731. Her captain, Robert Jenkins, had anchored for provisions in the harbor of Havana, Cuba. Suddenly the Spanish Coast Guard boarded the ship. There was a brief, furious skirmish, but the Spaniards were too many and too well armed. They captured the vessel, her crew and her cargo. Fandino, the Spanish captain, then **severed Robert Jenkin's right ear from his head**, following which, he courteously handed the ear to its former owner.

One year later, **with his desiccated ear wrapped securely in a leather pouch**, Robert Jenkins stood before a hushed Parliament and told his story. England promptly declared war on Spain.

The war was variously known as King George's War or The War of Austrian Succession. But most historians remember it as "**The War of Jenkins Ear**."

England's first priority was to appoint a commander who might decisively conduct strategic operations in the Americas, a vast distance from London. Prime Minister Robert Walpole chose an irascible, ex-member of Parliament named Admiral Edward Vernon.

Vernon was known for some eccentric habits, which had inspired a curious nickname. While topsides - no matter what the weather - he always wore a long coat made of a thick, coarse material which the French called *gros grain*. The British, unable or unwilling to pronounce it in French, called the material **grogram**.

Vernon wore that coat in heavy gales, in snowstorms, sleet, and hail. He also wore it at the peak of the Caribbean summer. Therefore, the sailors nicknamed their irascible and eccentric commander - "**Old Grog**."

This cantankerous admiral exhibited one other idiosyncrasy, not quite as appealing to his troops. In addition to crustiness, he was downright stingy. Nowhere was this more conspicuous than during the traditional happy hour, which every vessel of his Majesty's fleet diligently observed. Rum was the customary beverage, carefully stored in the ship's larder along with the food.

Old Grog did not relish the prospect of weekly drunken brawls on board his ship. Nor was he especially pleased at having to pay the price for rum - which came out of his budgetary allotment for all ship supplies. Therefore, he ordered his quartermaster to dilute the rum with water - a ratio of one part water to three parts rum. This infuriated the crew, but they could do nothing but carp and grumble - and rename the liquid refreshment after its author.

They called it **grog**, a name that has held to this day. In fact, after several pints of this libation one might actually become **groggy**. Such neologisms are a testimony to the resilience and innovativeness of the English language, and a durable monument to an obscure despot and his coat.

Old Grog is fortunately remembered for more than his intoxicating lexical contributions. There was still the War of Jenkins Ear to resolve. In 1739 Vernon and his men captured the Spanish town of Portobelo. This somewhat surprising achievement obliged Prime Minister Walpole to outfit an additional one hundred ships and place them all under Grog's tyrannical authority.

Then came Vernon's *coup de grace*. In 1741, he sailed into the Spanish harbor of Cartagena with 27,000 troops. They stormed the fort of San Felipe, but the Spaniards drove them back. During the following two months his army made several assaults on the fort. All failed.

Finally, they were forced to retreat. In England, Grog's brief glory following Portobelo subsided very quickly, eclipsed by this later deplorable failure, and the crusty old curmudgeon simply faded into Britannic oblivion.

There is an interesting side note to this obscure and less than momentous piece of history. During the battles at San Felipe, Old Grog had decorated a captain from the American colonies for exceptional heroism. That captain was Lawrence Washington of colonial Virginia, half brother to nine-year-old George Washington.

Shortly after the War of Jenkin's Ear, Lawrence Washington resigned from the British navy and retired. He returned to farm the plantation that had been left to him by his father. It was called Little Hunting Creek Estate. Lawrence Washington soon renamed the property to honor his former commander.

He called it Mount Vernon.

Old Grog had just moved from obscurity to perpetuity.

Libation and Auscultation

In 1846, Antoine-Joseph **Sax**, known to his friends as Adolphe, patented the instrument that bears his name: the **saxophone**. Those of us who cherish the syncopation, doo-wop, bebop, and jazz of people like Stan Getz, Coleman Hawkins, Buddy Tate, Sidney Bechet, John Coltrane, and Charley Parker, are forever grateful. Mr. Sax created his musical instrument using a single vibrating reed attached to a horn that has a conical bore and utilizes the standard fingering style of an oboe. The oboe, once characterized by Danny Kay as "an ill wind that no one blows good", gets its name from the fact that it is a soprano instrument made of wood. (French *haut* : "high" + *bois*: "wood" , a high-pitched wood wind. The French word haut is pronounced "oh", the bois sounds like "bwa" - thus, "oh-bwa", which eventually became oboe.) The root *haut* can be readily identified in **haughty**, someone who is insolent, conceited, or "high and mighty". *Haut* is also manifest in the borrowed French expressions *haute couture*: designers of "high fashion" (*couture* : "sewing"), and *haute cuisine*: "elegant food" (*cuisine*: "cooking").

In the 17th century a Benedictine monk shoved a cork into a fermenting bottle of wine, thus forcing the carbon dioxide bubbles to dissolve in the liquid. With this experiment he had created a drink that complements any haute cuisine , a "sparkling wine". In France, production of such wine is confined exclusively to the old province of Champagne, which explains the generic name for this bewitching beverage.

That monk, whose genius we toast, was cellarmaster of a monastery near Eparnay, France. At age 15 he had renounced the carnal world and entered the Benedictine order. Although he was blind, he possessed an uncommon sense of smell and taste, enabling him to distinguish subtleties of flavor and aroma. Several years ago, **Moet et Chandon**, the famous winery, named its finest champagne for this unpretentious monk, whose name was Pierre Perignon. The champagne is better known as **Dom Perignon.**

There are three grades of champagne, each depending on the sugar content. **Brut** has the lowest sugar concentration and is considered "heavy" or very "dry",that is, not sweet. (French *brut* from Latin *brutus* : "dull or heavy".) Champagne with a slightly higher sugar content is known as **sack** or **sec** from the French *sec,* which stems from the Latin *siccus*: "dry". The **sicca syndrome**, or keratoconjunctivitis sicca , derives from the same root. It is also called **Sjogren's Syndrome** and is usually accompanied by **xerostomia**. (Greek *xeros* : "dry" + *stoma* : "mouth". The copy machine invented in 1937 by a law student named Chester Carlson, takes advantage of a dry photographic process, which is why he called it the **Xerox**.) One need hardly state that "dry sack" is an egregious redundancy.

Henrik Samuel Conrad **Sjogren** was head of the Eye Clinic at Jonkoping, Sweden, in 1933, when he described his eponymous disorder in the Acta Ophthalmologica. He subsequently developed the technic for corneal transplantation, and became full professor of Ophthalmology at Goteburg University.

Champagne with the highest sugar content is called **doux,** which is French for "sweet", deriving in turn from the Latin *dulcis*, with the same meaning.

(**Dulcet** tones are sweet to the ears, and **Dulcinea** - "sweet one" - was the profligate beneficiary of Don Quixote's courtly affection.)

The original Benedictine monastery was founded in 529 at Monte Cassino, Italy, by **Benedict of Nursia**, known as the father of western monasticism. Members of this order wear a full black cowl and hood, which accounts for their sobriquet: "black monks". One of the most renowned Benedictines was **St. Augustine**, who sailed to England in 596 A.D. to convert the Anglo-Saxons to Christianity, and later became the first Archbishop of Canterbury.

In the year 1510, at the Benedictine monastery in Fecamp, France, a monk named Don Bernardo Vincelli created one of the oldest and finest liqueurs ever to grace the human palate. The liqueur is named Benedictine, after the order itself, and was created "to the greater glory of God". Each bottle carries the stamped initials **D.O.M.** - "*Deo Optimo Maximo*" - "for the most good and great God".(The name Benedictine itself derives from the Latin *Benedictus* : "blessed", which descends in turn from *bene* : "well" + *dicere*: "to speak", that is, to speak well (of) or to bless. One sip of Benedictine will convince you the liqueur retains its invocation.)

The Benedictine monastery at Monte Cassino was located at the very crest of the mountain, some 1700 feet above sea level, and was on the main route from Naples to Rome. During World War II, the monastery was the scene of fierce combat as allied troops, under the command of General Mark Clark, attempted to advance from their Anzio beachhead northward to Rome. Regrettably, on February 15, 1944, allied bombers destroyed the entire abbey and most of the town, in the famous **Battle of Cassino**.

From the Renaissance to the present, people have hoisted their glasses of Dom Perignon, Benedictine, sherry, and other alcoholic drinks, to **toast** each other - wishing success, happiness, long life, and good fortune to their friends. This ritual began in the 16th century, and derived from the practice of placing croutons of toast in the bottom of each glass. The toast, which was often spiced, was believed to add flavor to the drink - and also to adsorb acrid impurities within the alcohol.

Sherry is a fortified blend of wine that originated, and continues to be produced, in the Spanish city of Jerez (full name Jerez de la Frontera - "of the frontier" - referring to its proximity to the existing Moorish border.) The city began as a Roman colony named for Julius Caesar - **Caesariana** - which ultimately evolved to Jerez. The British could not easily pronounce Jerez, so they called its famous product "sherry".

The word **alcohol** is derived from the Arabic *al koh'l,* which was originally a smooth antimony powder used by women to darken their eyelashes. Eventually, medieval alchemists applied that term to any fine, velvety powder. Soon it came to indicate the vapors of fine steam arising from a boiling liquid.

Alcoholic libations are concocted by thermal vaporization. Fermentation first creates a mixture containing alcohol, water and other chemicals. Since the boiling point of ethanol is much lower than water, as the solution is heated the alcohol evaporates quickly, leaving the other ingredients behind. The vapors produced (now specifically known as **alcohol**) are then condensed as they flow through a cooling element, and the purified alcohol drips slowly into a collecting flask. The entire process is called **distillation** from the Latin *destillare*, which in turn derives from *de* : "from" + *stillare*: "to drop". The final product is obtained - drop by drop.

Sometimes the distillery is simply called a **still** - which has often given rise to new careers such as **bootlegging** - emanating from the practice of smuggling illicit hooch within the legging of boots. (**Hooch**, incidentally, stems from the Hoochino Indians, a Tlingit tribe that lives in southern Alaska, which unfortunately learned the art of distillation from their white oppressors.)

In ancient Greece, wine was carried in large jars that had a narrow neck and two handles. These urns were known as *amphora*, from *amphi* : "on both sides" + *pherein* : "to carry". They were often large enough to hold 40 quarts or more, and required two winebearers to carry them.

Ages ago, someone blew across the top of an empty amphora. (Coke bottles had not yet been invented.) A deep, bass musical tone was produced. Eons later a French clinician named Laennac heard such a sound arising from a tuberculous cavity. He called it **amphoric breathing.**

It sounded like a saxophone.

Patronymic Patois

Muhammad ibn-Musa al-Khwarizmi was born in what is now the city of Khiva, Uzbekistan. At the time, around 780 A.D., it was called Khwarizm, from which his family obviously took their surname. He was an intelligent lad who eventually became a noted astronomer, as well as librarian to the Caliph of Baghdad.

Although he wrote several volumes on astronomy, he is mostly remembered for his works on mathematics. Indeed, he was the first to use the term **al jabr** to signify the mathematical integration of symbols into numerical equations, for the purpose of solving complex arithmetic problems. (Arabic *al*: "the" + *jabr*: "bone-setting", that is, the science of setting fractured bones. **Al jabr** meant precisely that until well into the 16th century.) Khwarizmi employed **al jabr** in a metaphorical arithmetic sense, a connotation that has endured long after its original intent. Today we call this numerical discipline: **algebra.**

That has proven quite fortunate for many patients, since orthopedists would otherwise practice "algebra" - and who knows what mathematicians might be doing.

Al-Khwarizmi is also remembered for having contributed another term to mathematical science, one derived from his name. The term is: **algorithm**. (Al-Khwarizmi was corrupted by Westerners to <u>algorism</u> and then to <u>algorithm</u>.) Computer scientists, in particular, have adopted this particular model of arithmetic computation.

Arabic names, such as our protagonist's above, are rather confusing. Knowing that the prefix *al* refers to "the house of", as in al-Khwarizmi: "the house of Khwarizmi", is helpful. The term *ibn* means "son of", as in <u>Abdul Aziz ibn-Saud</u> (the first king of Saudi Arabia) - here it signifies the "son of Saud".

Many Hebrew names bear the designation *ben*, as in <u>David Ben-Gurion</u>, the first prime minister of the state of Israel (1949-1953), and <u>Eliezer Ben Yehudah</u>, a distinguished Lithuanian scholar. The Hebrew *ben* is identical to the Arabic *ibn*, both meaning "son of".

The identification of one's surname by paternal reference is, of course, not confined to the Semitic tribes of the mideast. English and American names such as John<u>son</u>, Ben<u>son</u>, Jack<u>son</u>, Eric<u>son</u>, Robert<u>son</u>, and Thompson (Thomasson) should serve as eloquent reminders that each man is his father's son.

Not to be thwarted, the Scots and the Irish herald the birth of their male heirs as MacDonald, MacArthur, MacDougal, etc. (or tachygraphically: McDonald, McArthur, McDougal). *Mac* in Scottish-Gaelic, of course, means "son of". However, the O'Briens, O'Rourkes, O'Haras, O'Caseys, O'Keefes, O'Kellys, and O'Neills need not recoil with remorse - since the **O** in their name correspondingly indicates "descendent, in Old Irish".

In Russia we find such luminaries as Igor Fyodorovich Stravinsky (composer), Andrei Dimitrievich Sakharov (physicist), Aleksandr Feodorovich Kerensky (revolutionary), Yuri Alekseyavich Gagarin (cosmonaut), and Boris Fydorovich Godunov (Czar), who each bear testimony and fidelity to his paternal progenitor. *Vich*, in Russian, obviously denotes: "son of".

This patronymic mania does not, however, obtain in every corner of the globe. Early Hindu culture, for example, boasted names that were matriarchal in evolution. Such derivations are called **metronymic**.

Of course, a logical consequence of patronymia would be that children must have a different surname from their parents. Consider Eric, son of Magnus. Eric's surname would naturally be Magnusson. Eric's son Lief, however, would have a different surname: Ericson. This could become quite confusing to those historians who research family pedigrees.

Fortunately for electoral polls, market research, and pie charts, this quandary was recognized, and at some point the family master and overlord, that genius of organization and control, decided to retain his surname as the historical family name, to be applied to all his descendants.

A daughter of patronymy suddenly had an embarrassing problem. Up to that time, for example, Lief's sister had been called Grindle Ericdotter. Henceforth, however, she would be known as Grindle Ericson. Nevertheless, women swallowed their collective pride, and moved ahead with their lives. (Another arrow in the quiver of feminine revolution.)

Surnames are a fairly recent development in human history. Up to the 13th century very few men possessed such a luxury. However, as society became increasingly complex, as the population grew, many individuals held the same given name. It became essential to distinguish between them for military, legal, civic, punitive, demographic, and other purposes.

Several adopted the surname of their profession. Thus arrived the Tailors (Taylors), Bakers, Carpenters, Coopers, Butlers, Gardeners

(Gardners, Garners), Weavers, Smiths, Barbers, Turners, and Millers, along with dozens of others.

Some were identified by their own personality or habitus. So we have Mr. Small, Black, White, Goodbody, Simon, Fox, Wolf, Short, Fine, Sharp, Witty, Silver, Keen, Spacey, etc. More than a few took the name of their village or city. Entire families of York, Oxford, Paris, Lincoln, Stafford, Kildare, Waterford, Mayo, Down, Sutherland, Ross, Kent, Dorset, and Washington, to name but a few, owe their lineage to an accident of natal geography.

The term **surname** derives from French *sur* from Latin *supra*: "above or extra" + *nom*: "name" - a name that is above or additional to one's given name. (Surtax and surcharge are comparable idioms, indicating "a tax or charge above and beyond another tax or charge". I assume that's something like "preboarding" an airplane.)

If you think about it, there is something about a surname that whispers of mud huts, cobblestone streets, Tamerlane, the Tower of London, and the Black Death.

But without your special cognomen you might still be known as Charles the Simple or Richard the Lion-hearted. Instead, you have become Charlie **Babbitt** or Richard **Couer de Leon**. Or perhaps even - Richie **Corleone**.

Of course, there are still a few who preserve their celebrity with but a single label like "Madonna", or "Liberace", or "The Donald". Some are even identifiable by initials alone, like L.B.J., F.D.R., or even O.J.

Stick to patronyms.

Political Potpourri

At age 30 he was a Marxist and the editor of Italy's leading socialist daily : *Avanti*. He was also a major factor in the decision by which Italy entered World War One on the side of the Allies.

Unfortunately, the Communist party opposed his position on that issue. He, therefore, resigned from that faction and formed his own party. In the 1932 edition of the *Enciclopedia Italiana* he described his new party's political philosophy. The essay he wrote was entitled: "*Dottrina del fascismo*" - the Doctrine of **Fascism**.

His name was Benito Mussolini, and he was the architect of Italy's Fascist Party.

His party's name was inspired by ancient Rome. In those days, a woodsman usually carried his axe tied within a bundle of sticks. The Latin word for bundle is *fasces*, and the thong which tied the bundle together was called a *fascia.*

The symbol of Roman authority eventually became a picture of an axe tied to a cluster of straw. **Lictors** brandished this emblem as they cleared the way for the chief magistrate. (Lictors were lesser officials whose title derived from the standard which they carried. Latin: *lictor* from the verb *ligate*: "to tie", another reference to the thong or strap with which the bundle was fastened.)

Aesop, the 6th century B.C. fabulist, had once written a parable about sticks. The legend described the ease with which a single branch could be snapped in two, but the effort required to break a collection of them. In usurping an Aesopian fable, as well as an ancient Roman symbol, the Fascists declared to the world that they were "bound" together. In their unity was their strength.

From the verb *ligare* we obtain ligate, ligament, and ligature. The verb is also hidden in such words as religion and obligation ("ties" that bind us morally).

In medical parlance, the word **fascia** ("bundle") initially described a narrow fibrous band. Later its meaning was expanded to indicate a sheet of connective tissue. A **fasciculus** is "a little bundle" - as in bifascicular and trifascicular heart block and muscular fasciculations. It is also found hidden in words like fascination - a word suggesting "spell**bound**".

Fascism has disappeared as a manifest system of government, at least for the time being. However, there are other political derangements that still persist.

For example, there are aristocracies, plutocracies, theocracies, and democracies. **Democracy** evolved from the Greek *demos*: "the people." Such words as demography (the statistical or graphic study of populations), and demagogue (Greek *agogos*: "leader", i.e. "leader of the people"), are also derivatives. An epidemic is something that is prevalent "among (Greek - *epi*) the people". The epidemiologist is one who studies (Greek - *logos*: "the study of") these disorders.

A **monarchy** (Greek *monos* : "alone" + *archein* : "to rule") is a society ruled by a king or queen. **Anarchy** (Greek *an*: "without") is a community without a ruler or government.(An Archbishop is the chief or ruling bishop (from *archein* : "to rule"). A **bishop**, parenthetically, stems from Greek *epi* : "upon" + *skopein* : "to look" - as in microscope. A bishop is one who "looks upon" or supervises a diocese. The **Episcopal** Church, which is ruled by bishops, has thus acquired its name. (Incidentally, the bishop's **miter**, a tall ornamental cap with front and back peaks, was thought to resemble the left atrio-ventricular heart valve by early prosectors. Therefore, we have the origin of **mitral valve**. From Latin *mitra*: "the headdress worn by the ancient Jewish high priests")

A hierarchy is a government ruled by the church (Greek *hieros*: "sacred or holy"). **Hieroglyphics**, for example, were the sacred pictographic writing of ancient Egypt, inscribed by the high priests. (Greek *gluphein*: "to carve".) An **oligarchy** (Greek *oligos*: "small or few") is a government in which the ruling power belongs to very few people. **Phenylpyruvic Oligophrenia** comes from the same etymological root. (Greek - *phren* : "mind"). Also known as phenylketonuria, or PKU, this genetic disorder results from the inability of the cells to metabolize phenylalanine to tyrosine, resulting in mental retardation. These tragic patients, in other words, are intellectually deficient or "small-minded".

And we're back to politics.

Republic derives from the Latin *respublica,* which derives from *res*: "things" + *publica*: "public". That is, "public things" or matters pertaining to the public interest. (The famous - or infamous - legal phrase *res ipsa loquitor*: "the thing speaks for itself", may be familiar to you.)

Intermittently, a form of madness overwhelms certain governments. In the U.S. it is a phenomenon that recurs quadrenially. We refer to it euphemistically as an **election**. (Latin *electus* the past participle of *eligere* : "to pick or choose".) **Candidates** are selected by party **caucus** and spend a great deal of time and money going on the **stump** to convince the average **voter** to cast his **ballot** for them. **Polls** are conducted to ascertain whom we will undoubtedly elect. These statistically elegant polls reassure us that we will not find an unexpected surprise in the morning newspaper. (See Truman, Harry S. 1948.) We always elect a **president**, several **senators**, and many **congressman** - usually an order of magnitude more than are necessary or useful. These folks are subsequently **inaugurated**.

Candidate is from Latin *candidatus* : "clothed in white". In ancient Rome, those who aspired to public office wore white togas to proclaim their purity. (see Agnew, Spiro, and Nixon, Richard; etc.,etc.)

Caucus derives from an early political and social club in Boston known as the "Caucus Club". One of its members was John Adams. The name caucus stems from an Algonquin Indian term *caucauasu* : "counsellor". This contribution to American politics appears to represent the sole political function permitted our Native Americans, until they were reluctantly granted the right to vote by an act of congress in 1924.

To go on the **stump**: stems from the fact that tree stumps were abundant in colonial America, the result of clearing the land for agriculture. A politician simply had to step onto one of these natural platforms to launch into his speech. (To be "stumped", that is puzzled or frustrated, derives from the difficulty experienced by those who attempt to remove the arboreal remnants, which tenaciously cling to their birthplace.)

Vote derives from Latin *votus* : "a vow". A vote cast, therefore, is a vow of support for the candidate. (Would that it might be reciprocal.)

Ballot is from Greek *ballein* : "to throw" (from which ball is derived) The ancient Greek method of voting was accomplished by tossing a marble into a container. A white ball represented a vote for the nominee, a black ball a vote against. Thus the origin of "blackballing" someone. The word **bullet** also comes directly from *ballein*. This may account for the confusion between bullets and ballots, occasionally seen at some elections.

Poll is from the Dutch *polle* : "crown of the head". Thus a poll is, strictly speaking, a head count. Ornithologists use the term in such designations as the Blackpoll Warbler and the Redpoll, birds with either a black or reddish crown. To "poll a tree or bush" is to cut the top off. Cattle are also "polled", their horns being removed. **Tadpoles** are "toad heads". Anyone having observed these aquatic larva will attest to the aptness of the name. (**Polliwogs** are "wiggling heads",another apt designation.)

President is from Latin *praesidere* : "to preside". This in turn derives from *sedere* : "to sit". Naturally, the president must sit at the head of the table to run his meeting. He is, therefore, the quintessential chairman, or chairwoman, or chairperson (which, I surmise, is neither man or woman).

The word chair comes from Latin *cathedra* and designates the throne of a bishop, or any seat of high authority. To speak *ex cathedra* is to lecture with the prerogative that comes from one's special office or rank. (The **cathedral** itself is the building in which the bishop ordinarily sits on his chair.)

Senator derives from the Latin *senex*: "old or ancient", as in senescent. It implies that the Roman senate was composed of older, wiser citizens. Not so in every senate or in every country.

In Greek, the word for old is *presbys* as in **presbyopia** or **presbycusis**, both frequent consequences of aging. The **Presbyterian** Church is guided by an ecclesiastical council and a governing body of older members.

Congress is from Latin *congressus*: "a meeting, a coming together, or social intercourse." It may also connote sexual intercourse. (None of that, of course, relates to members of our federal government.)

Inaugurate stems from the Latin *auger* - which , in turn, derives from *avis* : "bird" + *gerere*: "to handle" - that is, to handle birds. In ancient times, special diviners, mystics and oracles prophesied the future by killing and dissecting birds, the entrails of which provided clues to the future. Before a major event - a battle, coronation, or portentous regal decision - the **augur** would be called to exercise his predictive skills, usually to prophesy a victory for the incumbent sovereign or ruling junta. Some fortunetellers, perhaps reluctant to handle entrails, resorted to the flight pattern of living birds to divine the future. These were "bird watchers", or *avis* (bird) + *spicere* ("to observe"). From this idiom, Latin *auspex* was derived, which ultimately resulted in the term **auspicious**).

An inauguration is, unfortunately, not always an auspicious occasion.

Baseball

On April 12, 1861 the stillness of Charleston, South Carolina was shattered by mortar fire. Confederate troops under General Pierre Gustave Toutant Beauregard, fired the first round in a long, bloody war. Thirty four hours later Robert Anderson, the Commander of the garrison at Fort Sumter, surrendered. Among his 85 men was an artillery officer who had ordered the first retaliatory shots fired by northern troops. His name was Captain Abner Doubleday.

Today, we remember Abner Doubleday, not for this abbreviated niche in our nation's archives, nor for his subsequent advancement to the title of Major General of Volunteers, nor for a distinguished military career during which he fought at Antietam, Bull Run, Fredericksburg, and Gettysburg.

In fact his most celebrated accomplishment had occurred well before the outbreak of civil (or uncivil) hostilities. It happened in the summer of 1839, while serving as instructor in a military prep school at Cooperstown, New York, when Abner Doubleday introduced his students to a new game. The game was based on the English pastime known as **rounders**. Doubleday called his version - **baseball**. Historic records clearly show that he had neither invented the game, nor the rules by which it was played.

Nonetheless, it served the interest of those major league moguls who ultimately took control of the sport, to promote that fiction. In 1939 - at the alleged centennial of baseball's origin - the Baseball Hall of Fame was dedicated in Cooperstown, New York. To earn a shard of historic respectability, its promoters submitted a Civil War hero - Abner Doubleday - as its "inventor". Leo Tolstoy once remarked: "History would be a wonderful thing - if it were only true."

Alexander Joy Cartwright, a surveyor who sometimes played for a baseball club called the New York Knickerbockers, was the man who actually designed the rules for baseball. The date was June 19, 1846. The place was the Elysian Field at Hoboken, New Jersey. His Knickerbockers were soundly trounced by the New York Nine, 23 to 1 - but that contest was the first baseball game played under modern regulations.

In 1869 the first professional team was established. They were called the Cincinnati Red Stockings and their manager was Harry Wright, a local jeweler and center fielder. Harry was paid the bountiful sum of $1200 that year. Seven years later, on February 2,1876, at the Grand Central Hotel in New York City, the National League was formally created. Charter members included Boston, New York, Chicago, Philadelphia, Hartford, St.Louis, Cincinnati, and Louisville.

The opening game of the very first National League season saw Boston edge Philadelphia 6-5. It was on April 22, 1876. Two months later - on the morning of June 25, 1876 - a company of 264 men from the U.S. Seventh Cavalry, under the command of General George Armstrong Custer, entered the valley of the Little Bighorn River. The story of baseball was temporarily eclipsed.

Baseball patois has entered the language of America from the first cry of: "Play Ball!" To have "two strikes against you", to be slightly "off base", to "go to bat" (for a cause), to "keep pitching", and to "keep your eye on the ball" - all owe their origin to its joyful jargon.

Which of us is unfamiliar with the technicality of a stolen base, a double, a triple, a round-tripper, a force out, double play, double header, spitball, beanball, squeeze play, shoestring catch, pop-up, fly ball, pitchout, pick-off, or foul ball???

A few terms, however, do require some explanation, and here I should like to offer a potpourri of baseball words that have piqued my curiosity.

In 1872 a shortstop named Dickey Pearce, playing for the Brooklyn Atlantics, reached out with his bat and gently butted a pitch. The ball rolled slowly toward third base and stopped. Before the astonished third baseman could recover sufficiently to field the ground ball, Pearce had safely crossed the first base bag. A "butted ball" instantly became an offensive weapon. However, as wit' many woids, the nasal Brooklyn twang altered the word to **bunt**.

In 1901 the American League was created. A johnny-come-lately, they have been known as the **junior circuit** ever since. The National League is, of course, the **senior circuit**. The American League was initially comprised of eight teams : Chicago (managed by Clark Griffith), Boston, Detroit, Philadelphia (owned and managed by Connie Mack), Baltimore, Washington, Cleveland, and Milwaukee.

The (old) Baltimore Orioles were organized in the 1890's. Under third baseman-manager, John McGraw (later of New York Giants fame), they became the most surpassing team in early baseball history. Unfortunately, the franchise folded. Baltimore, bereft of major league baseball, patiently waited 50 years. Finally, the St. Louis Browns moved their team east to start the 1954 American league season - as the regenerated Baltimore Orioles. (Take heart Brooklyn and Washington!)

John McGraw and his teammate "Wee Willie" Keeler invented the **Baltimore chop** - a ball deliberately struck so as to be driven into Baltimore's hardened infield. The impact caused the ball to carom high in the air, hanging up long enough for the speedy batter to reach first base, before an infielder could throw him out.

The term **rookie** comes from the word "recruit", and did not become part of baseball vernacular until after World War One. A **fan** derives from someone who is "fanatic" about the game.

The **Grapefruit league** stems from spring training camp, which used to be held exclusively in the citrus state of Florida.

Bull Durham is the name of a chewing tobacco. It was common for the old baseball parks to display a huge billboard ad with the bright red, green, and brown bull, emblematic of the product. In this same section of the ball park, enclosed by a fence and at some distance from the playing field, one usually found the relief pitchers. Is it any wonder that some baseball wag, seeing the relievers warming up in front of the Bull Durham sign, enclosed within their own little corral, should coin the phrase **bullpen**?

A **rhubarb** is a heated, fulminating, window-rattling argument, usually conducted between an umpire and one of the teams, but occasionally involving both squads, and often resulting in the expulsion of one or more players. The term was popularized by Red Barber, who was arguably one of the finest baseball announcers (for the now extinct Brooklyn Dodgers). The word rhubarb is actually a theatrical term. The actors in Hollywood's angry crowd scenes were instructed to mumble "rhubarb, rhubarb, rhubarb....." in order to simulate the sound of an irate mob.

Bleacher seats are found at the upper reaches of a ball park, the area usually occupied by the true baseball afficionados. Not covered by roof or dome, the wooden benches are exposed to the weathering rays of sunlight, and so they bleach.

No game would be complete without a cadre of **umpires** to arbitrate, explain, clarify, and disambiguate closely contested calls. Their word is final - they are the law. Umpire derives from French *noumper*: "odd or not even" - a reference to a third person who referees and adjudicates a dispute between two parties. *Noumper* evolved from Old French *nonper* that, in turn, derives from Latin *non*: "not" + *par*: "equal". After incorporation into Middle English, and through a linguistic process known as juncture loss or false splitting, "a noumper" became "an oumper". Eventually, it emerged as "an umpire". (Juncture loss may also be noted in the word **apron**, which began its life as the Latin *mappa,* evolved through Old French *nape*: "tablecloth", and became *naperon.* Eventually, "a naperon" became "an aperon".

In 1887, Peter Finley Dunne, a youthful reporter for the Chicago Evening Post, sat in the press box at Sox Stadium, and composed his baseball column for the next day. A left handed pitcher was on the mound and Dunne searched his mind for a colorful phrase to describe the scene. Sox Stadium, like all open baseball parks, was designed so that the batter faced east directly at the opposing pitcher. This was done so that the afternoon sun would never shine directly into the batter's eyes. (Of course, the outfielders - especially the center fielder - always look toward the west, requiring those fancy flip-down sunglasses.) As the pitcher also faces west toward the batter, a left-hander's arm must arc through the south, as his pitch is made. Thus Dunne coined the term **southpaw**.

The list of baseball terms is almost endless. Our language has been infinitely enriched by them. Find out for yourself. Take in nine innings. Bring a friend. Buy some hotdogs. Maybe you'll get lucky. Maybe it'll go into **extra innings**. As Jack Norworth and Albert von Tilzer wrote in 1908:

"Take me out to the ball game, take me out to the park. Buy me some peanuts and Cracker

Jacks, I don't care if I never get back......"

Eponyms III

Hodgkin's Disease, discussed elsewhere, is one of many medical eponyms. However, eponyms are hardly peculiar to medicine. The word itself comes from Greek *epi* : "upon" and *onyma* : "name".It refers to proper nouns, names of people or places, (often lower-cased by history) that have been applied to ordinary articles or objects.

In other essays I focus rigorously on the myriad examples which comprise, in large measure, our own medical patois. But here let's examine some representative eponyms that are familiar to a general, non-medical audience.

Guppies , for example. Those inch long, brightly colored fish, usually found swimming in fresh water aquaria - are named for R. J. Lechmere Guppy of Trinidad, who discovered them. **Monkey wrenches** are another example. They were named for the mechanic who invented them. His name was Charles Moncke and he worked for the firm of Bemis and Call of Springfield, Massachusetts.

The **ferris wheel** was invented by George Washington Ferris in 1893.The **saxophone** by Antoine Joseph Sax - with financial assistance from his good friend Hector Berlioz. **Silhouettes**, shadowy profiles of people,were designed for fun by Etienne de Silhouette, a good friend of Madame **Pompadour**, who had him appointed the Controller General of France in 1759.(She, too, has been eponymized , her name referring to a style of haircut popular in the 1940's and early 1950's - remember Ed "Kooky" Byrnes of "77 Sunset Strip"?)

Chauvinism - often thought to be the creation of the women's movement - is actually derived from Nicolas Chauvin, a soldier in Napoleon's Grand Army. After suffering multiple wounds in battle, Chauvin was retired on a small pension. But he so idolized the Little Corporal that even after Napolean's ignominious defeat, and for the remainder of Chauvin's life, this fanatic preached only of the infallibility of his hero, and the magnificence of France. A chauvinist was, initially, a provincial, flag-waving jingoist, filled with blind patriotism. Sexist males are a recent modification.

The most famous circus acrobat of the 19th century, the man who perfected the aerial somersault, is not remembered for that accomplishment. He is recognized for the clothes he wore during the performance. His name was Jules **Leotard**. And the men who invented the lighting that lit the stage for his act were German brothers John and Anton Kliegl. Their name was too hard to pronounce, so the light they developed is known as a **klieg** light.

During our Revolutionary War, a captain in the Virginia militia from Pittsylvania County organized an impromptu court to rid his territory of Tories and other scoundrels. Unfortunately, the justice dispensed was often as injudicious as it was swift. The rogues were abruptly hanged. The captain was William **Lynch**, and the punishment now bears his name.

One hundred years later and an ocean away, another captain delivered his name to eponymic posterity. The English Earl of Erne owned a huge estate in County Mayo, Ireland, therefore he hired a captain to supervise his tenant farmers. Unfortunately, a series of crop failures, culminating in the famine of 1880-81, made it impossible for the tenants to pay their rent. Instead of sympathy, however, the captain responded with brutal retribution - evicting several of the farm families. The farmers and their friends retaliated. No one spoke to the captain. He could not buy food or clothing at the local shops. He was totally ostracized from the community. All his servants left him. Finally he surrendered, quietly taking his family and leaving the country.

His name was Captain Charles Cunningham **Boycott**, and his name is now associated with that tactic.

In 1850, a Texas lawyer who was a hero of the Mexican War, found himself the recipient of a herd of cattle as payment for his services. However, the lawyer was not a rancher and quite uncertain about how to manage this reimbursement. He moved them to an island in the Nueces River, just off the Matagordo Peninsula. A winter drought virtually dried up the river, and many of the unbranded cattle wandered across and settled on neighboring ranches. Once there, they did not remain unbranded very long.

The lawyer was Samuel Augustus **Maverick** - and his name, too, has found its way into our semantic history.

Several foods owe a debt of gratitude to proper names. Consider **Bibb** lettuce - named for its developer ,an amateur gardener named John B. Bibb. Or the **Bing** cherry - for a Chinese man who cultivated the tree in Oregon in 1875. Or the **sardine** - named for the island around which it thrives - Sardinia.

Consider **bourbon** - which was first produced in Bourbon County, Kentucky. And **booze** itself - named after its distiller E. S. Booze of

Philadelphia - who poured the contents into a bottle shaped like a log cabin, with his name on the label.

When you think of eponymic food can one ignore **beef Strogonoff**, or **beef Wellington**? Count Paul Strogonoff, a 19th century Russian diplomat, and Arthur Wellesley, the first Duke of Wellington, are responsible for these delights.

And can one possibly overlook the contribution rendered by that 18th century libertine and gambler - John Montagu? Refusing to leave the gambling table to eat, he ordered his servant to bring him a slice of roast beef between two pieces of toasted bread. Thus did the Earl of **Sandwich** provide us with that culinary delight.(As the head of the British Admiralty during Captain James Cook's famous voyage, he was honored to have the newly discovered Sandwich Islands named for him as well. It is now known as Hawaii.)

Chicken Tetrazzini was prepared especially for the Italian diva Luisa Tetrazzini. And **melba toast** developed and named for the Australian opera star Dame Nellie Melba. So, too, a dessert of peach ice cream with raspberry sauce: **peach melba**.

Another dessert, the delectable **praline**, that crunchy sweet almond roasted in sugar, which is so popular in New Orleans. It was invented by the Comte du Pressis-Praslin in honor of his guest, King Louis XIV.

In the early 1800's a Presbyterian minister, convinced that refined white flour was not good for health, urged thousands of his followers to bake bread and crackers with unrefined, whole wheat flour. The products were named after the preacher - Sylvester **Graham**.

However, we not only find eponyms to eat, we find them to wear as well. **Argyle** socks, named for the Duke of Argyle and his Scottish clan, were originally green and white diamond patterns. Today only the diamond pattern is preserved, but the socks are multi-colored.

On October 25,1854, Major General James Thomas Brudenell, bedecked in his bright red and blue uniform, led his 11th Light Dragoons into the teeth of a heavily armed Russian force at Balaclava, Crimea. This was the famous "charge of the Light Brigade", made famous by Alfred Tennyson's epic poem. The General wore his woolen vest to protect against the biting cold. That vest's reputation has outlasted the memory of its wearer, who was also known as the seventh Earl of **Cardigan**.

The man who gave the order for that famous and catastrophic charge was the Commander of all British Forces, General Fitzroy James Henry Somerset. He, too, wore a distinctive outfit, a loose-fitting coat with sleeves that stretched to his neck. This was, in part, to disguise the fact that he had but one arm - the other having been removed by field surgeons at the battle of Waterloo. The memory of Somerset's exploits - like Brudenell - has evaporated with the mists of history. But his coat, especially those unique sleeves, are monuments to his memory. He was also known as the First Baron **Raglan**.

Hats have eponymic origins as well. Consider an early 19th century Englishman named Edward Stanley. He was fond of horses and horse racing. He also habitually wore a round bowler hat. In 1870 Mr. Stanley instituted an annual race for three year olds at Epsom Downs. The contest soon became a British favorite, whose popularity continues today. In fact, the race had become so renowned, that in 1875 the idea was imported into the United States, has flourished, and is now part of the famous Triple Crown. Mr.Stanley was also known as the 12th Earl of **Derby**. The English and Kentucky varieties - as well as the hat - all derive from his name.

Then there's the man who first recognized a cowboy's need for a large hat to screen him from the sun. So in 1885,in the city of Philadelphia, he started manufacturing 10 gallon, soft - brimmed, high-domed cowboy hats. The cowboys called them "John B's". The man was John Batterson **Stetson**.

Other apparel have also carried the imprimatur of the eponym. **Tuxedoes** were first developed in Tuxedo, New York. **Bloomers** were developed by Mrs.Elizabeth Miller in 1850 but created such controversy that she and her associates were not allowed to attend church services and were threatened with excommunication. This warning, however, failed to intimidate feminist Amelia Jenks <u>Bloomer</u> who wore them provocatively and often - and was rewarded for her valor by their nominal designation to posterity.

B.V.D., is simply the abbreviated (pardon the pun) name for the company that created and manufactured them - Bradley, Voorhees and Day.

Botanists, too, have had a field day with eponym. Consider the following partial list:

Wisteria,Fuchsia, Poinciana,Magnolia, Begonia, Camellia, Poinsettia,Dahlia,Forsythia, Gardenia, and Zinnia.

They were named for: Casper **Wistar**, M.D.(anatomy Professor at the University of Pennsylvania), Leonard **Fuchs** (German physician and botanist - basic Fuchsin, a reddish-purple aniline dye is also named for him), M.de **Poinci** (governor of the West Indies in the 1600's), Pierre **Magnol** (French physician and botanist), Michel **Begon** (royal commissioner of Santo Domingo in the 17th century), George Joseph **Kamel** (Jesuit missionary and amateur botanist), Joel Roberts **Poinsett** (American Minister to Mexico in 1825), Anders **Dahl**_(Swedish botanist), William **Forsyth** (a very well-known Scottish horticulturist), Alexander **Garden**, M.D. (Scottish-American physician who was an ardent tory. He left South Carolina to return to England during our Revolutionary War), and Johann Gottfried **Zinn**, M.D. (who authored the first anatomical atlas of the eye, became the first director of Botanical Gardens in Gottingen, Germany, and for whom the central retinal artery is named.)

Zoysia grass is also eponymic, having been developed by Austrian botanist Karl von **Zois**.

The list of common words derived from proper nouns is astonishing and continues to grow. Our automobiles, including the **Buick**, **Cadillac**, **Chevrolet**, **Pontiac**, **Ford**, **Oldsmobile**, **and Chrysler** - are all named after people. The **Diesel** engine is named for the German engineer who invented it - Dr.Rudolf **Diesel**. The **Rolls-Royce** is named for two people: Sir Henry **Royce**, who designed the car, and Charles Stewart **Rolls**, champion race car driver (who later became the first Englishman to die in an airplane accident).

In 1901 the Daimler company named their fashionable automobile for the daughter of their largest car dealer. Her name was **Mercedes** Jellinek.

And the cognoscenti of the N.R.A. should be able to tell you that Colt, Browning, Smith and Wesson, Thompson, Derringer, Winchester, Carbine, Maxim, and Mauser are all eponyms for their inventors. The Gatling gun - or "gat" as Bogart liked to refer to it - was one as well. So,too,was the <u>Minnie Ball</u> - made famous during our Civil War. It was invented by a French army captain,Claude Etiene **Minie**.

Indeed, **shrapnel** itself was invented by British Second Lieutenant Henry Shrapnel in 1783. (**Flak**, in case you were interested, is not an eponym. It is a German acronym devised during WWII. It stands for **<u>Fl</u>**ieger **<u>A</u>**bwehr **<u>K</u>**anone - "flier defense cannons".)

William Shakespeare asked : "What's in a name? That which we call a rose, by any other name, would smell as sweet." Eponyms, names of forgotten people and ancient places, word fossils of mankind's yesterday, will surely embellish and enrich our speech forever.

As we pontificate, babble, prattle, mutter and mumble - we often bear silent, unrecognized witness to those lives which might otherwise have passed forgotten.

Handiwork

The state medical society of Maryland is formally known as "The Medical and Chirurgical Faculty". Several years ago, someone suggested we parenthetically explain what the Medical and Chirurgical Faculty is by adding the clarification: "Medical Society of the State of Maryland". A physician seated next to me at a meeting leaned over and whispered : "What the hell does Chirurgical REALLY mean?"

Cheirourgos is the Greek word for "surgery". It stems from *cheir* : "the hand" + *ergon* : "work" - therefore, it is "handwork" or work performed by one's hands. (Things that surgeons do best.) Thus the Medical and Chirurgical - or surgical - Faculty.

Cheir may be found in several words, such as **chiropractor** - one who practices (a type of treatment) by using his hands. The Chiropractor performs a **manipulation** (*manus*: Latin for "hand"). One may also note an obsolescent specialty: the **chiropodist** - one who treats hand and foot (Greek :*pous*) diseases. Today they are called **podiatrists**, having now limited their practice strictly to feet. The mammalian order *chiroptera*, which includes the familiar bat, owes its taxonomy to the same source (*cheir*: "hand" + *pteron*: "wing" - it is an animal with a "winged hand". A **helicopter** is from Greek: *helix*: "spiral" + *pteron* : "wing". The "spiral wing" refers to the rotating propellers.)

Ergon, the Greek word for work, is found in **energy** - Greek *en*: "at" plus *ergon* : "work", that is, to be "at work". In fact, you may recall that the unit of work accomplished by one dyne acting through a distance of one centimeter is called an **erg**.

As noted, the Latin word for hand is *manus*. When one **manufactures** something we make it (Latin: *facere*) by hand. And the instruction **manual** describes how the hands must execute that task. That is precisely the reason we refer to them as **handbooks**. Incidentally, old **manuscripts** were actually written (Latin: *scribere)* by hand, a subtle form of manual labor.

The French word *manouvrer* means "to cultivate the land" (by working with the hands). Years of lexical evolution has resulted in the word **manure,** literally the stuff our hands must maneuver to fertilize the soil.

The **manubrium**, which is the widened, upper sternal shield, appeared to some creative prosector to look very much like the handle of a sword. Therefore, it was named - *manus*: “hand” + *habere*: “to hold” - to hold in the hand, as a sword **handle**. The caudal portion of the sternum is called the *xiphoid* which, in Greek means “like a straight sword”. In Latin it is called the *ensiform* process (*ensis*: “sword” + *forma*: “shape” - “sword-shaped”). The name of the body of the sternum is seldom recalled. It is known as the **gladiolus** from Latin *gladius:* “sword”.

All **gladiators** will grasp these penetrating observations.

The **Gladiola**, a tropical member of the Iris family, has funnel-shaped flowers arrayed on one side of the stem, and a few sword-shaped leaves from which it obviously derives its name.

Pediatricians owe their name to the Greek words *paidos*: “of a child” + *iatros*: “physician”, that is, a children's physician. (**Iatrogenic** refers to disorders that are “caused by” (Greek: *genic*) physicians.)

Orthopedics arises from Greek *ortho*: “straight” plus *paidos*, that is, to “straighten a child”, obviously a reference to correcting bony and cartilaginous deformities in youngsters. It is not related, as some have thought, to the Latin word *pes*: “foot” - the genitive of which is *pedis* : “of the feet”.(As in **pedestrian**: “one who walks”, or **pedal**: something that is “operated by feet”.)

A **pederast** (from Greek *paidos*) indulges his grotesque carnal obsessions with (male) children. A **pedagogue** (from *paidos* + *agein*: “to lead”) - that is, “to lead, or teach, a child” - is an educator. An incongruity results, however, when teachers are too **pedantic**. An **encyclopedia** derives from Greek *enkyklios*: “circular” + *paideia*: “instruction of children in the circle of arts and sciences”.

Words derived from Greek *pous* or Latin *pes*, both of which refer to feet, are myriad and occasionally camouflaged. From the Greek we find such items as **tripod** (Greek - *tri*: “three”, something that has three feet), **octopus** (Greek- *octo*: “eight” - having eight feet), **platypus** (Greek - *platy*: “flat”, the animal is obviously flat-footed), **polyp** (Greek - *poly :* “many” + *pous* – “many-footed”), and **podagra** (*pous* + *agra*: “seizure” - that is, “foot seizure”, or gout).

From Latin we derive **impediment** - something that ensnares or entangles the feet, **expedite** - something that frees one who is caught by the feet, and **pedunculated** - the narrow stalk of a tumor, which appears to be attached “by a foot” to its host. The **piedmont** region of a region lies at the foot of its mountains (Latin *mons*: “mountain”), and one’s **pedigree** is a genealogical chart whose lines connect generations of relatives.

To some creative French author it appeared to resemble the *pied de grue* - the “foot of a crane”.

Anchors Aweigh

The Greek word for ship or boat is *naus*, from which we derive most **nautical** terms. The Greek term for "seasickness" - *nausia* - comes from this root and, slightly altered, has become **nausea** . Roman society subsequently converted *naus* into the Latin *navis*, which still meant "boat", and a host of English words were created including **navy, navigate**, and the **navicular** bone. This small bone of the human wrist resembled a "little boat" to an imaginative early prosector. Some anatomists also call it the **scaphoid** bone, preferring the older Greek derivation (*skaphe*: "small boat" + *eidos*: "like, or resembling", that is, "like a small boat".)

A few physicians may remember a freshman mnemonic that recalls the carpal bones: "Never lower Tillie's pants, mother might come home". When decoded, it translates to the navicular, lunate, triangular, pisiform, greater multangular, lesser multangular, capitate, and hamate - the eight carpal bones of the hand.

Incidentally, the word **mnemonic**, which means "memory aid", originates from the Greek goddess of memory, **Mnemosyne**. (Parenthetically, she had once enjoyed a memorable evening with Zeus, and subsequently gave birth to the Nine Muses - her contribution to mythologic memorabilia.)

The **nave** of a church, which is the main part of the building between the side aisles, is aptly named because of its architectural resemblance to a ship. But the **navel**, that dimpled remnant of one's last attachment to serenity, has a very different etymology. It comes from the German *nabel*, meaning "a central point".

(A **Navel orange** is a seedless fruit named for the umbilical-like depression at its apex.)

There are many words that come from nautical jargon. The **bow**, or front, of the ship is from Swedish and is analogous to **bough**, the branch of a tree, which it resembles. The **stern**, or rear, of a ship is a foreshortened rendering of an Old Norse word meaning "the steering end" (of the boat), where the rudder is found.

The derivation of starboard and port is quite interesting. Viking ships were equipped with a large, flat paddle that projected from the right hand side of the ship (as one faces forward). These paddles were used as side rudders to steer the ship, and were called *stoeranboards* in Old English. This meant "steering board", and through linguistic evolution has become **starboard**.

Because the steering board protruded from the right side, all boats had to dock on the left side. In Old English that side became known as the **hladanboard** - or "loading board" side - which was soon contracted to **ladenboard**, and finally to **larboard**, partly to rhyme with starboard. This should explain the famous sea chantey: "Tis larboard and starboard you jump to the call, Yo-ho blow the man down..."

However, during periods of severe weather, as the captain would order his men either "to larboard" or "to starboard", the roar of wind and waves often rendered his commands indistinguishable. The resulting confusion often caused navigational catastrophes. Therefore, in the 17th century, the British Admiralty changed the term larboard to **port**, and the potential confusion was avoided. The port side became the loading side, the dockside, the side that faced the port city - the left hand side of the boat, as one faced forward.

The hull of an old-fashioned wooden ship was constructed of wooden planks that were separated by seams. The seams were known as **devils** in 16th century naval parlance. This term was derived from the French *diable*, and probably arose because the seams were hellish to maintain. They often leaked and constantly had to be re-sealed with hot tar or pitch. The French verb *payer* meant "to apply hot pitch". Therefore, when the ship docked for repairs at some suitable island, there was **the devil to pay**.

This job was most difficult when the main, or keel, seam was involved. At such times, the crew had to tilt the ship onto one side in order to expose the seam. Then, a few very unlucky sailors, dangling precariously from the side, endeavored to fill the gaps with boiling tar, while the ship rolled and lurched on the incoming whitecaps.

Of course, as the sailors dangled there in terrified suspension, they were both literally and figuratively **between the devil and the deep blue sea**.

Vivé la France

The game of tennis originated in France, evolving from a 12th century game known as *Jeu de Paume* : "the palm game". (tennis - from French *tenez:* "receive!", a term that is used to warn an opponent prior to a serve). The scoring expression "love", as in "40 - love" (40 to nothing), is from the French *l'oeuf*: "the egg". In France, as in this country, "nothing" is often characterized by a zero, and a zero looks very much like an egg. Baseball pitchers hurling a shutout are said to be throwing "Goose eggs" at the other team. *L'oeuf* became anglicized to "love". Thus *quarante - l'oeuf* is "40 – love".

In 1789 the French nobility and the clergy (the First and Second Estates) conspired to sell France's entire granary stores to foreign countries for a handsome profit. Unfortunately, the French peasants and bourgeois (the Third Estate) were acutely starving. (*Bourgeois*: "shopkeepers, the middle class", which emanates from Latin *burgus* : "castle or fortification". The German word *burgh:* "fortified place or town", and the English **borough**, have a similar derivation.)

Third Estaters were not enraptured at the prospect of a national famine. Therefore, they demanded a vote in the *Estates-General* (National Assembly) that would have assured an equitable distribution of grain to all French citizens. Hearing of this, the aristocracy canceled the entire legislative session.

Third-Estaters collectively left the parliament building and assembled at a nearby tennis court, where they convened their own session. At that meeting, which became known as the *Serment du Jeu de Paume*, "the Tennis Court Oath", they solemnly promised each other that they would not cease until France had achieved a democratic constitution. Three weeks later, July 12, 1789, citizens of the Third Estate attacked the Bastille. The French Revolution had begun.

A prominent member of the National Assembly during those frenetic days was a French physician whose name was Joseph Ignace **Guillotin**. Joseph had come from the small town of Saintes, and at age 51 was elected to office from his district. In the assembly, Guillotin had spoken passionately about a "new machine" by means of which death sentences might more expediently be accomplished. The instrument to which he referred had actually been invented by another physician, Dr.

Antoine **Louis**, and was originally called a "**louisette**". In his remarks to the assembly Guillotin said : "the victim will feel nothing but a slight sense of refreshing coolness on the neck. We cannot make too much haste, gentleman, to allow the nation to enjoy this advantage".

Shortly thereafter the Reign of Terror began under the sadistic command of Robespierre. Louis XVI was executed in January 1793. His queen - consort, Marie Antoinette, was dispatched ten months later. Before it was over, more than 15,000 people had been executed, including the inventor of that macabre instrument of death, Dr. Louis himself. Somehow, Dr. Guillotin escaped and fled his native land, but his name had become forever chained to the executioner's tool: the **Guillotine**. His family sought anonymity by changing their name, but could never quite erase the repugnance attached to it.

However, as France danced maniacally to the rock'n roll of a new democracy, French physicians began a hesitating minuet with some new ideas of their own, concepts that would establish French medicine as preeminent in the 19th century. A partial list of some names should convince even the most passionate skeptic: Phillipe **Pinel**, Rene **Laennac**, Armand **Trousseau**, Pierre-Adolph **Piorry**, Guillame **Duchenne**, Jean-Martin **Charcot**, Prosper **Meniere**, Pierre-Paul **Broca,** and Guillame **Dupuytren**.

Perhaps the most popular surgeon of that era was Dominique-Jean **Larrey** (1766-1844). He had written clinical descriptions of trench foot, scurvy, and the use of gastrotomy feeding tubes. Larrey's prowess at nimble, expeditious surgery was legendary. Once, during Napoleon's disastrous Russian campaign, Larrey had performed over 200 amputations in a single day!

But his most significant contribution to medicine was the introduction of horse-driven wagons, which were used to transport stretchers to the battlefront, and carry the wounded back. These were called "mobile hospitals" - *hopital ambulant*.

After a time the "*hopital*" was dropped, and they simply became **ambulances**.

Microbe Hunters

In 1260, the Yuan dynasty was founded by Kublai Khan, the grandson of Genghis Khan. On his fabled trip to the Far East, Marco Polo met Kublai Khan. Shortly thereafter Polo, his father Niccolo, and uncle Maffeo, entered the Great Khan's service as foreign advisers to the Mongols.

On returning to Italy in 1295, Polo described his incredible odyssey, which encouraged Venetian merchants to begin exploring trade with Cathay. (Tartar word for China). Unfortunately, in 1333 the Black Death emerged from the agrarian, oriental villages. Very soon thereafter, Genoese merchants returning to Italy with treasures of silk and furs, were ambushed by rapacious Tartars. These bandits launched a siege at the Crimean trading post of Caffa, trapping the merchants. But during the assault, plague ripped through the Tartar hordes, weakening them and forcing their withdrawal. Prior to their evacuation, the Tartars catapulted their dead over the wall into Caffa, thus infecting the Italian merchants who became inadvertent human vectors for the spread of bubonic plague into Europe.(Bubonic: from Latin *bubo*: an enlarged, inflamed lymph node).

Rats are the primary reservoir for this disease, particularly *Rattus rattus*, the common house rat. Rat fleas (*Xenopsylla cheopsis*), which feed upon the infected blood stream of their murine host, become engorged with *Yersinia pestis*, the responsible bacterium. The fleas then infest their human hosts, transmitting their deadly charge. (Yersinia, named for Swiss bacteriologist **Alexander Emil Jean Yersin**, are gram negative, non-motile bacteria of the family Enterobacteriaceae. This family also includes the Genus *Salmonella*, *Escherichia*, *Proteus*, and *Serratia*. (*Yersinia pestis* used to be called *Pasteurella pestis* when I was younger, but taxonomists must make a living somehow.)

Italian physicians quickly realized that isolating plague victims would render great protection to the community. They ultimately sealed the port of Venice to all ships for a period of forty days, beginning March 20 1348. Three years later, travelers entering any Italian city would be isolated for the same period of time. This was the first use of the **quarantine** in medical history. (Quarantine - from Italian *quarantina,* which represents a contraction of *quaranta giorni*: "forty days".)

Xenopsylla cheopis ia also the arthropod vector of the rickettsial infection **typhus**. (Typhus, from Greek *typhos*: "vapor or smoke", implying that the disorder is somehow transmitted by noxious fumes. This etymology is parallel to that for **malaria**, Italian for *mala aria*: "bad air", again implying that the illness was somehow induced by the miasmic vapors arising from swamps.)

Typhus is one of a number of diseases caused by rickettsiae, which are intracytoplasmic, gram negative, pleomorphic organisms, named for the American pathologist Howard Taylor Ricketts. Mites, ticks, lice, and fleas each have a special role in promoting individual rickettsial infections. *Rickettsia prowazekii* is responsible for epidemic typhus, as well as **Brill-Zinsser** disease, a milder recurrence of this disorder. (The genus prowazekii is named for Stanislas J.M. von Prowazek, a German zoologist who first identified the offending organism. Nathan **Brill** was a New York City physician who first recognized the recrudescent form of typhus in 1898. Hans **Zinsser** was an American bacteriologist who first suggested that these patients were simply carriers of typhus, who occasionally experienced flareups of a milder nature. Zinsser is noted for having written "*Rats, Lice and History*", a history of the men and women who dedicated their lives to solving the mystery of infectious diseases.)

Both Ricketts and von Prowazek died from typhus, thus fulfilling Koch's postulates, and earning them the eponymous gratitude of posterity.

Other infectious disease terms have had an interesting origin. *Influenza* is Italian for "influence", since astrologers of medieval times believed that the disease was under the influence of the stars.

Brucellosis, from the genus *Brucella*, is named for **Sir David Bruce**, a British military physician who first described the disorder. (It is also known as **Malta Fever** since it was prevalent on that island, and had been isolated from the spleen of a soldier stationed there, who had died of the disease.)

Botulism, caused by a neurotoxin secreted by *Clostridium botulinum*, owes its derivation to the Latin *botulus*: "sausage", prompted by the belief that contaminated sausages were poisonous. Not far from the truth.

Shingles comes from the Latin *cingulum* : "a belt , or girdle". The term obviously describes the distribution of the lesions. *Herpes* is Greek for "creeping eruption". *Zoster*, also Greek, means: "girdle".

A rose by any other name.

There's Never Been A Good One

The Latin participle for "speaking" is *fans.* A small human who had not yet spoken, was called an **infant** - *in*: "not" + *fans*: "speaking". The original meaning was soon expanded to include youngsters, whether they could actually speak or not. Thus the female heir to the Spanish throne was referred to as the **infanta**.

In the Middle Ages, a noble French lad who had not yet reached knighthood was called an *enfant.* In Italy he was known as an *infante* and it became his job to walk behind his knight's intrepid steed, carrying the warrior's armor. An entire garrison of these children was known as an *infanteria.* Thus was born the foot soldier, the dogs of war, the **infantry**. Perhaps the ineffable wartime tragedies, which they witnessed, had rendered them speechless. War does that sometimes.

On the other hand, war causes us to fashion new terms, to create its own distinctive jargon.

For example, there were the Parthians who, from 247 BC to 224 AD, ruled the region that we now call Iran. One of their great kings was Mithridates who commanded a superb army, and developed some superior new battle tactics. For instance, in battle his cavalry would appear to be routed and begin a wholesale retreat. But as the enemy pressed forward, the fleeing Parthians would suddenly turn in their saddles and fire their arrows, killing or wounding many of their astounded opponents. This was known as a **Parthian shot** - and over years of lexical evolution, the term has become a **parting shot.**

Mithridates himself has earned a meager place in our lexicon. Ruthlessly, he had deposed his Queen Mother and quickly became a most unpopular monarch. Even within his own castle, and among his most trusted aids, he feared for his life. Therefore, he began consuming small amounts of various poisons in the belief that he could build a tolerance to their lethal effects.

After a failed war against the Roman legions that angered his own troops, there followed a bloody revolution and a *coup d'etat.* Mithridates, dreading a tortuous death, attempted suicide - but he had developed a tolerance to the poison and it did not work! The king was "hoist by his own petard". He was subsequently impaled on a sword by one of his loyal disciples. (The technique of inducing tolerance to poison by administering small and gradually increasing amounts of the substance, is now called **Mithridatism.**)

Incidentally, the Greek word for bow was *toxon.* (toxology: "the study of archery".) In battle, Greek warriors coated their arrows with a drug known as *toxicon pharmakon* - "the poison of the bow", in a manner similar to the Indians of South America who use curare - tipped arrows when hunting game. The venomous substances used by the Greeks soon became known as **toxins**, borrowing the poison from the weapon itself.

To become **intoxicated** is literally to become poisoned or drugged, and is most often applied to alcoholic debauchery. After all, doesn't the bartender request that you "name your poison"?

Modern chemistry has characterized alcohol as an organic compound that contains an hydroxyl group. In addition to our favorite ethyl alcohol, we have methyl (wood) alcohol, butyl alcohol, isopropyl alcohol, glycerol, ethylene glycol (antifreeze), etc. Certain physiologic sterols such as **cholesterol**, **ergosterol** (precursor of vitamin D), and vitamin A (**retinol**), are also alcohols. (Cholesterol was named because it is present in most gall stones. Thus Greek *chole*: "bile" + *stearin*: "fat" + "**ol**" to indicate its alcoholic character.)

Cholesterol is chiefly composed of a complex carbon ring structure known as the cyclopentanoperhydrophenanthrene nucleus. Estrogen, testosterone, cortisone, and other hormones resemble cholesterol in that they are also mainly composed of this nucleus, but lack the alcoholic hydroxyl group. So they are known as "**cholesteroid**" (Greek *oiedes*: "like, or resembling") that is, a substance that reminds you of cholesterol. Soon these chemicals were simply called "**steroids**". (digitalis glycosides are also steroids, which undoubtedly accounts for the tender breast enlargement seen as an occasional side effect of the drug.)

Hoist by one's own petard refers to the petard, an explosive, cone-shaped apparatus filled with gunpowder, which was detonated by a fuse. In ancient warfare it was used to blast holes in a defensive wall, or to demolish the gates of a castle. Unfortunately, the infantryman whose job it was to plant the bomb, often became part of the fireworks. Quality control was not as extraordinary as it is today.

Incidentally, the term petard derives from French *peter*: "to fart". This droll metaphor undoubtedly suggested the sound of the explosion, although some of us believe it actually referred to the commanding officer who ordered the maneuver.

The **musket** was an early firearm, which evolved in Spain during the 1500's. It was a smooth bore shoulder-fired weapon. To load the gun, a soldier first poured gunpowder into the muzzle, followed by a two-ounce steel ball. In the earliest models, lighting a match and holding it to the gunpowder pan ignited the powder. These were known as **matchlock rifles**. They were superseded by the more sophisticated **flintlock rifle** invented in 17th century France. A spring-loaded hammer or striker was connected to a trigger. On squeezing the trigger the hammer was released striking a piece of flint and showering the gunpowder with sparks, which caused the requisite explosion needed to propel the metal ball. Occasionally, the trigger mechanism failed, releasing the hammer too soon. This caused the gun to **go off half-cocked**. Moreover, if the gunpowder were damp (as could occur during a heavy rainstorm) the gun would not fire at all. This resulted in the well-known admonition **to keep your powder dry**. Furthermore, there were occasions when the powder would ignite, but then fizzle out without firing the shot. This was known as **a flash in the pan**.

The Dutch expanded the distal end of the musket, filling it with several smaller metal balls. When the gun fired, the shot scattered widely over a very short distance - the first shotgun. They called it a **donderbus** (*donder*: "thunder" + *bus* : "gun"). The accuracy of this weapon was laughable, thus prompting the British to coin a pun, deriding the weapon as a "**blunderbuss**".

Our own Civil War enlarged the language, even as it diminished the population, which spoke it. The first American **Admiral**, David Farragut, was commissioned in 1866. (Admiral from the Arabic *Amir a'Ali*: "high leader".) Other familiar military terms such as **AWOL**, **draftee**, **ensign**, **pup tent**, and **war correspondent** were born during this war of national shame. The famous **Springfield rifle** was developed and built in Springfield, Mass.- and the equally renowned **Sharps' rifle** was designed by Christian Sharps. The men who used it proficiently came to be called **sharpshooters**.

World War One further expanded our combat patois, adding much bureaucratese and military gibberish. On May 7 1915, **U-boats** sank the British ocean liner Lusitania off the Irish coast, with the loss of 1200 passenger lives. (German *unterseeboot* : "undersea boat" or "u"- boat., for short). In 1918, **Big Bertha** shelled Paris from 75 miles away. "Big Bertha" was the mocking and derisive name applied to a giant cannon manufactured by the famous Krupp steel works, the owner of which was a rather corpulent German dowager - Frau Bertha Krupp von Bohlen und Halback.

We developed all sorts of interesting names to call the Germans and their army: **Hun** (modeled after Attila himself), **boche** (French contraction of *allemond* + *caboche*, which became *alboche*: "German Cabbagehead". The term was later shortened to boche). **Heine** (short for "Heinrich", a common German name), **Fritz** (scornful nickname for "Friedreich", another common German name. The word was later incorporated into a disdainful expression of incompetence: to be "on the fritz"). **Jerry** (German helmets resembled chamber pots that, in England, were known as "jerries"), and **Kraut** (short for "sauerkraut", a German dietary staple).

The British soldiers were known as **Tommies**. This evolved from a sample English recruiting form in which the applicant was named "Tommy Atkins", synonymous with our "John Doe". The Brits were also known as **limeys** - from the early practice of feeding English sailors lime juice as an antiscorbutic on long ocean voyages. (Latin **scorbutus**: "to wither and grow ill". In 1754 Dr. James Lind,a British naval surgeon,published "A Treatise On Scurvy" in which he recognized the value of citrus fruit in the prevention of the disease. At the time more sailors were dying of scurvy than were being killed in combat. However, it wasn't until 1795 that the Royal Navy ordered lemon or lime juice for all ships of the fleet. Scurvy disappeared abruptly - and British sailors have been "**limeys**" ever since.)

Doughboys, as our soldiers were called, stemmed from the large buttons adorning their uniforms, which resembled dumplings or fried sweet corn cakes of the same name. American soldiers were also known as "**Joes**", (a generic American nickname) and since they were Government Issue - "**G.I. Joes**", and then simply "**G.I.'s**". They wore metal identification tags around their necks, which resembled dog licenses hanging from a collar - hence "**dogtags**".

Khaki uniforms became standard during WWI (Hindi: *khaki* - "dust covered"). The men dug long, deep ditches that were called **trenches** , from which arose such famous expressions as "**trench knife**" and "**trench coat**", as well as several diseases including "**trench foot**", "**trench mouth**", and "**trench fever**".

But the true mercenary in this global conflict was a respiratory virus - **Influenza**. Emerging from Spain in 1918 it swept the world, becoming a true **pandemic** (Latin *pan*: "all" + *demos*: "people"). The first outbreaks occurred thousands of miles apart - Boston, Mass., Brest, France, and Freetown, Sierra Leone. At Camp Devens in Massachusetts the first case occurred on September 12, 1918. Eleven days later 12,604 men had become gravely ill. In contrast to most influenza epidemics, this one killed young as well as old. Within the camp morgue, bodies "the color of slate" were stacked like cordwood. The lungs filled rapidly with a thin, bloody exudate. Eyewitnesses described young men who turned blue before them and died in less than 48 hours. Colonel William Henry Welch, a pathologist who had been the first Dean of Johns Hopkins Medical School (1893-1898) - and who had discovered the gas gangrene bacillus - was sent to Camp Devens to direct medical operations. There was very little he could do to stem the plague.

When it was over 675,000 Americans - including 24,000 soldiers - were dead. Worldwide totals have been estimated at 22 million deaths, although that figure is surely conservative. (India alone had 12 million dead - with estimates of as high as 30-40 million).

Our total battle deaths in WW1 were 53,513.

The name **influenza** originates directly from Italian *influenza* : "influence". It was a disease, which the ancients believed was entirely under the influence of the stars.

Perhaps they were correct.

Evil Days

Medieval calendars typically classified two days each month as "days of evil". On those days, it was unwise to begin any enterprise, for bad luck would almost surely result. The days were known in Latin as *dies mali* (*dies*: "days" + *mali*: "of evil").

By the middle of the 15th century, *dies mali* had become "**dismal**", and any inauspicious or unlucky day was called, redundantly, "a dismal day".

As the world quietly turned, the meaning of dismal gradually mutated from "bad" or "evil" to merely "gloomy", "dreary", or "woeful". The days of evil had moderated.

The Latin *dies* has found its way into other familiar expressions, in some of which it was quite evident, in others rather camouflaged. *Medius* (Latin: "middle") plus *dies* combined to form *meridies*, which became **meridian**: "middle of the day", or mid-day, or noontime. *Ante* (Latin: "before") plus *meridies* thus became "before mid-day, or **A.M**. and *post* (Latin: "after") *meridies*, **P.M**.

The geographic meridian on which you are currently located, is your longitude. On this line, the sun is at its zenith and is precisely south of you at noon (local time) each day. The Prime Meridian is at 0 degrees longitude, passes through Greenwich, England, and by international convention is the point of reference for every longitude in the world, as well as for world time. Since there are 1440 minutes in a day (24 hours X 60 min.), and since the earth encompasses 360 degrees of circumference, it follows that each degree of longitude equals 4 minutes of time. 15 degrees of longitude, therefore, equals one hour of time. The world time zones are referenced to Greenwich Mean Time (GMT) at 0 degrees longitude. (In military patois this becomes known as **Zulu Time** - the "Z" in Zulu denotes the "Z" in zero longitude. For example, "1800 Zulu" equals 6 PM Greenwich Mean Time.)

Circa (Latin "around") plus *dies* combine to form **circadian**: "that which lasts for around a day". Circadian rhythms, such as our sleep cycle, the secretion of endogenous cortisol, or the timing of myocardial infarctions, thus fluctuate around the clock.

A **quotidian** fever is one that recurs on a daily basis (Latin *quot*: "as many as" + *dies*: "daily"). Double quotidian fevers manifest two febrile spikes daily and are occasionally symptomatic of tuberculosis, gonococcemia, or leishmaniasis.

Prescriptions are written for **B.I.D.** (Latin *bis*: "twice" + *in*: "per"), **T.I.D.** (*ter***:** "three"), **Q.I.D.** (Latin *quater:* "four"), or **Q.D.** (Latin *quaque***:** "every" + *die*: "day").

From *dies* stems the Latin *diurnalis* ("of the day" or "daily"). Something that has a **diurnal** variation, changes during the 24 hour day. Diurnal, however, may also refer to something that only occurs during daylight hours - an animal, for example, which hunts exclusively during daytime - as opposed to a nocturnal hunter.

From Latin *diurnalis* the French word *jour* evolved, as well as the Italian *giorno,* both of which mean "**day**". Whether one shouts *bon jour* or *buon giorno* - it's all the same - "good day". In Spanish, of course, it's *buenos dios***.**

A **diary** reflects daily events in the writer's life. So, in fact, does a **journal**. And when the president of an organization stands before his lectern and requests a motion to **adjourn**, he is in reality calling for the assembly to recess until a future date - *ad jour*: "to a day". (That day is usually a standard meeting time, which has all ready been scheduled. The motion to adjourn has the highest priority of any main motion, with exception of a motion to adjourn to a specific time. To adjourn *sine die* is to recess the meeting "without a date" to reconvene.)

To keep track of our days, humans have cleverly invented clocks. These have **dials** - from Latin *dies* through *dialis*: "daily". Clocks often measure the duration of a **journey**, which may take days.

The latter half of dismal (*mal*) has evolved from the Latin *malus*: "evil" or "bad", which gives us a legion of words, such as **malevolent**, **malady**, **malnourishment**, **malodorous**, **malabsorption**, **malice**, and that father of all evil, **malpractice**.

Petit mal is a "small" illness or malady (French: *petit malade*), whereas **grand mal** is a "large" one. **Malaria** derives from Italian *mal*: "bad" + *aria*: "air", from the primitive belief that the disease was induced by inhaling the miasmic air of nearby swamps.

A **malapropism** is a word that is used inappropriately. It derives from the French *mal* plus *a propos*: "to the purpose", and emanated from **Mrs. Malaprop**, a character in **The Rivals**, a 1775 play written by Richard Brinsley Sheridan. Mrs. Malaprop frequently muddled words that sound alike, and would offer such profound observations as: "If I reprehend anything in this world, it is the use of my oracular tongue, and a nice derangement of epitaphs".

Mal de mer is a direct borrowing from French: "sickness of the sea". *Mer* stems from Latin *mare*: "sea", as in **marine** and **maritime**, and may be recognized in **mermaid**. Interestingly, **nausea**, the typical consequence of *mal de mer*, stems from the Greek *naus*: "ship" and *nautes*: "sailor", pelagic roots that may also be found in terms like **nautical** and **astronaut** (Greek *astron*: "a star". Astronauts are metaphorical "sailors of the stars"). Clearly ancient civilizations were cognizant of the effect that the sea produces on one's balance, sense of well-being, and gastrointestinal tract.

For those of you who are superstitious, the following are the original *dies mali* ("evil days") of medieval calendars:

January 1 and 25; February 4 and 26; March 1 and 28; April 10 and 20; May 3 and 25; June 10 and 16; July 13 and 22; August 1 and 30; September 3 and 21; October 3 and 22; November 3 and 28; December 7 and 22.

One might almost envision a Roman dramatist writing play about these pernicious dates. The title might have been: "*Dies mali in Lapis Niger*".

Figure it out.

Eponyms IV

Eponyms are fascinating peeks into history. (Greek *epi*: "upon" + *onyma*: "name". An eponym is a term, which derives from a proper name, such as **Bright's Disease**, or **Hodgkin's Disease** (both discussed elsewhere). Eponyms - forgotten lives and faceless names - condemned to serve forever as humble, undistinguished common nouns.

Medical jargon is replete with examples, it is one of the profession's most endearing eccentricities. However, this idiosyncrasy is not merely confined to medical terminology. Consider, for example, the case of a Frenchman who became a German engineer. He sought to develop an engine, which would outperform the steam engine of Watts. In 1892 this German engineer patented his engine, and spent the rest of his life struggling to introduce it to the world. No one listened. In 1913, while crossing the English Channel, the inventor disappeared. He was never seen again. Only after his death did the world recognize that his engine incorporated a pivotal advance in machine design. Unfortunately, **Rudolph Diesel** never realized the triumph of his own genius.

There is also the tale of Queen Artemisia, whose husband ruled Caria around 400 BC (Caria was an area within Anatolia, now part of Turkey. Among its citizens were the famous Thales, Anaximander, and Pythagoras.) After her husband's death, Artemesia commissioned a magnificent burial chamber. It was built of marble with Ionic colonnades resting on a tall base surrounded by sculptured lions. At the summit there was a large pyramid with 24 steps leading to a magnificent chariot. The structure became one of the "seven wonders" of ancient civilization. It became indelibly associated with its only resident - King **Mausolus** - and ultimately culminated in the mysterious and haunting term : mausoleum.

Nevertheless, medicine still retains the title: "the mother of all eponyms". **Felty's Syndrome**, for instance, described by Augustus Roi **Felty** in 1924, is characterized by splenomegaly and pancytopenia, in patients with rheumatoid arthritis. Dr. Felty was a second year medical resident at Johns Hopkins when he wrote that paper. Unfortunately, his academic career was all too brief. He was obliged to return to Hartford, Connecticut to help his ailing father in General Practice. After 30 years in practice, Felty retired, and in 1964 he died of a stroke. But his eponymic disease endures.

Most medical eponyms are readily identified. **Bright**'s and **Hodgkin**'s diseases represent classic examples - as do **Babinski**'s sign, **Parkinson**'s Disease, **Huntington**'s Chorea, and **Raynaud's** Syndrome. However, there are several medical eponyms whose derivation from proper names is not quite so obvious.

For instance, a Y-shaped anastomosis that includes the small intestine is called a **Roux-en-y**. It is named for a Parisian surgeon who first described the procedure in 1908. His name was **Jean Charles Roux**.

Anatomic terms often bear the names of those who initially described them. **Gabriele Fallopio**, who described the oviducts that bear his name, originally expected to enter the seminary. Fortunately for us, Vesalius persuaded him to undertake a medical career. In 1551, Fallopio succeeded the great Vesalius to become Professor of Surgery and Anatomy at the University of Padua.

Fallopio's contemporary, **Bartolomeo Eustachio**, was his chief rival. In 1562 Eustachio described the small tubes that connect the nasopharynx to the middle ear. He was also the first to describe the adrenal glands, and he produced a remarkable set of 47, anatomical drawings that includes a spectacular illustration of the sympathetic nervous system, and of the valve guarding the entrance of the inferior vena cava into the right atrium. It became known as the **Eustachian Valve**.

One hundred years later, the auditory tubes were named for Eustachio by another obscure "eponymogenist" (a neologism that I have just created, meaning "one whose name becomes an eponym"). His name was Antonio Maria **Valsalva**, and a forced expiration against a closed glottis carries the Valsalva epithet.

In 1898, a cytoplasmic network of tubules and vesicles was discovered by **Camillo Golgi**, who was already known for his description of the chrome-silver nitrate stain for nerve tissue. The cellular organelle was understandably named the **Golgi Apparatus**. In 1906, Golgi was awarded the Nobel Prize in Medicine/Physiology.

Other well-known anatomic features such as **Pacinian Corpuscles**, **Meibomian** and **Nabothian** cysts, and **Negri Bodies** are also eponyms, named respectively for **Filippo Pacini**, **Heinrich Meibom**, **Martin Naboth**, and **Adelchi Negri**.

Frederich Luer, a German fabricator of glass instruments, invented the **Luer lock syringe**. The syringe is often used to start intravenous infusions of lactated **Ringer's Solution** - named for the physiologist **Sidney Ringer**, Professor of Medicine at University College in London, who used it to preserve his isolated frog heart preparations.

The **Moro Reflex** - the famous "startle response" - seen in normal children 6 months of age or younger, was described in 1910 by the Austrian pediatrician, **Ernst Moro**, who had previously isolated the *Lactobacillus acidophilus* bacterium, and was the first to introduce intradermal skin tests for tuberculosis.

The **Queckenstedt Test**, compression of the jugular vein to test for subarachnoid blockage, was developed in 1916 by a German physician, **Hans Heinrich Georg Queckenstedt**. An army truck killed him on the last day of World War I.

Petri dishes, Somogyi units, Westergren sed rates, Snellencharts, Wood's light, Rorschach tests, Wheatstone Bridges, Trendelenburg positions, Kussmaul breathing, and Christmas factor are each lasting monuments to the people for whom they were named.

Perhaps, after all, they shall no longer be entirely faceless labels.

Germs

Ferdinand Julius Cohn was born in Breslau, Silesia (now a province of Poland) in the year 1828. Although his name is hardly a popular household word, he has earned a shard of immortality from one of the smallest of living organisms. Cohn was a contemporary of both Pasteur and Koch, and the three of them were responsible for the birth of a new science: **bacteriology**. It was Cohn who first suggested that bacteria might be classified by their shape into **bacilli, cocci, and spirilla**, and it was he who attempted the first taxonomy of those microscopic creatures.

A **bacterium** ultimately derives its name from the Greek word *bacterion*, which is the diminutive of *baktron*: "a small staff or rod". Disconcertingly, the bacterium known as a **bacillus** has a similar derivation. It stems from the Latin *bacillum*, which is the diminutive of *baculus*: "a little rod or stick".

The **coccus** comes from Greek *kokkus*: "grain or kernel", and was given its name by the famous surgeon Theodore Billroth in an 1874 essay entitled "*Untersuchungen uber die vegetationsformen von coccobacteria septica.*" (Billroth achieved international fame from his surgical procedures for peptic ulcer disease, which involved excision of the pylorus and anastomosis of the residual stomach to either the proximal duodenum - **Billroth I** - or to the jejunum - **Billroth II**).

The organism **Spirillum** emanates from Latin *spira*: "a coil".

The **Streptococcus** evolved from the Greek *streptos*: "twisted as in a necklace or chain" and the **Staphylococcus** derives from Greek *staphyle*: "a bunch of grapes". Each prefix identifies the typical microscopic appearance of these gram-positive animalcules.

The **Gonococcus**, on the other hand, springs from Greek *gone*: "seed", and arose from the erroneous belief that the urethral discharge in **gonorrhea** represented the efflux of semen. *Rheos*, the Greek for "flow", plus *gone*: "seed" thus meant "a flowing of seed or semen." The gonococcus, therefore, is named as inaccurately as the disease, which it engenders. A more descriptive term may occasionally be heard at street corners. Pimpled cosmopolites call the disease "**the clap**" - derived from a medieval French term for a red light district: *Le Clapier*. The lusty French have given it an even more practical name. They refer to gonorrhea as *chaude pisse* ("hot piss").

Latin *vibrare* means "to quiver", from which the genus **vibrio** secures its name, owing to the characteristic motion initiated by its single polar flagellum. It vibrates.

Cholera, the disease caused by *Vibrio cholerae*, can be traced to the Greek *chole*: "bile" + *rhein*: "to flow". The profuse, markedly dehydrating, diarrhea of cholera was believed to consist chiefly of flowing bile. Robert Koch was first to recognize that **vibrio** organisms were responsible for this infectious scourge, the tragic sequellae of which he had observed during a tour of India and Egypt. (Koch, renowned for having discovered the tubercle bacillus, was first to isolate the Anthrax bacillus and to develop a vaccine for its prevention, and is still celebrated for having established "Koch's postulates" - a rigorous and exacting method to prove the etiologic relationship of organism to disease. In 1905 he received the Noble Prize for medicine.)

Greek *kampylos* means "bent or curved". A genus of small, gram negative, bent rods was therefore named *Campylobacter*. One of these organisms - *C.fetus* - causes human dysentery. It used to be known as *Vibrio fetus* when I was young medical student, but taxonomists have to make a living too. (*Campylobacter pylori* was recently renamed *Helicobacter pylori*, and is now considered responsible for the majority of peptic ulcer disease. Greek *helix:* "spiral".)

The Greek god of the sea, **Proteus**, was the son of Oceanus and Tethys. It was alleged that he possessed knowledge of everything past, present, and future. Since he never divulged these secrets, one was forced to catch him at his noontime siesta, bind him securely, and compel him to reveal them. Proteus, however, was capable of assuming an infinite variety of shapes, and always escaped imprisonment. The aerobic, gram negative bacterium *Proteus* derives its name from that ancient mythological sea deity with its chameleon-like disguises.

Moreover, the overused and often painfully contrived term "protean" - as in "the protean manifestations of this disease" - also stems from that versatile and polymorphic Greek god. Such stereotypical medical expressions are often accompanied by other sophomoric phrases, such as "a well-developed Caucasian male". All such pomposities issue from an underdeveloped recognition of the prosaic.

Finally, one should acknowledge the substantial contribution to our professional idiom afforded by men and women who have devoted their lives to the study of germs. Terms such as Bartonellosis, Gram stains, Bilharziasis, Leishmaniasis, Chagas'disease, Borreliosis, Kawasaki's disease, Reiter's syndrome, Reye's syndrome, Negri bodies, Salmonellosis,

Shigellosis, Bordetella, Nocardia, Neisseria, Klebsiella, Brucella, Listeriosis, and Pasteurella - to list but a very few.

These derive respectively from: a Peruvian physician - **Alberto Barton**, a Danish physician - **Hans Christian Gram**, a German helminthologist - **Theodor Bilharz**, a British bacteriologist - **Sir William Boog Leishman**, a Brazilian physician - **Carlos Chagas**, a French bacteriologist - **Amadee Borrel**, a French bacteriologist - **Jean Hyacinthe Vincent**, a Japanese pediatrician - **Tomisaku Kawasaki**, a German bacteriologist - **Hans Reiter**, an Australian pathologist - **Ralph Reye**, an Italian pathologist - **Adelchi Negri**, an American veterinarian - **Daniel Salmon**, a Japanese bacteriologist - **Kiyoshi Shiga**, a Belgium bacteriologist - **Jules Jean Baptiste Vincent Bordet**, a French veterinarian - **Edmond Nocard**, a German dermatologist - **Albert Neisser**, a German bacteriologist - **Edwin Klebs**, a British bacteriologist - **Sir David Bruce**, a British surgeon - **Joseph Lister**, and the French chemist, co-founder of the science of Bacteriology - **Louis Pasteur**.

They have each found immortality in our words.

Unless the taxonomists get bored again.

Amo, Amas, Amat

Twenty years before the American revolutionary war, a child was born to an Austrian violinist and his wife. They christened him: Joannes Chrysostomus Wolfgangus Theophilus. His parents were named Leopold and Anna-Maria Mozart. As he grew older the young man rejected the cacophonic sound of his many confusing names, choosing instead the last two and renaming himself: Wolfang Theophile Mozart. The middle name meant "lover of God", from the Greek *theo*: "God"(as in theology) and *philo*: "loving" (as in philosophy - a lover of knowledge). Later, in deference to the prevalent custom of Latinizing names, Mozart changed Theophile into Amadeus. (*Amo*: "I love" + *deus* : "God"). If the young man had not been so considerate, the 1984 Academy Awards might have gone to "Theophile" - or worse yet to "Gottlieb".

Mozart, sadly, lived but 35 years before succumbing prematurely to typhoid fever (or possibly rheumatic fever, according to a recent article). Nonetheless, he had lived in an interesting era. The year of his birth was noteworthy for the publication of James Lind's treatise "On the Most Efficient Means of Preserving the Health of Seamen", in which Dr. Lind described his experiments with scurvy. Lind placed six pairs of patients on different diets to determine which food offered the most significant protection from the dreaded disease. His best results were obtained with oranges and lemons. When Captain James Cook made his historic expedition to the South Pacific (1772-1775), he followed Lind's advice. Cook's men each received an allotment of citrus fruit. No scurvy occurred.

In 1844 Parliament mandated a regular issue of lime juice to all seamen. From that date to this, British sailors have been known as "**limeys**".

During World War 1, scientists at the Lister Institute in London began a meticulous search for the antiscorbutic factor. (Latin *scorbutus*: "scurvy" which, in turn, derives from the Russian word *skorbnut*: "to wither or grow ill".) They soon recognized that this essential factor was a new and unfamiliar vitamin. Fat-soluble A and water-soluble B vitamins having all ready been described, the unknown element was named water-soluble "C". It was finally isolated in 1927 and synthesized in 1932.

The term **vitamin** stems from the early observation that an amine of nicotinic acid prevented Pellagra. It was, therefore, called "a vital amine" - which was soon shortened to "vitamine" by Casimir Funk, a Polish-American biochemist. Subsequent research demonstrated that not all "vital factors" were amines, therefore the final "e" was dropped and the word simply became "vitamin".

Other pivotal medical advances were developed during Mozart's brief lifetime. In 1760, a physician in Padua, Italy published a study, which was acclaimed by the medical community. It was titled: "*On the Seats and Causes of Disease*". Giovanni **Morgagni** thus introduced the anatomical concepts, which founded the science of pathological anatomy. And in 1762, Nils von Rosenstein, a Swedish physician, wrote "*The Diseases of Children and Their Remedies*", thus establishing the specialty of Pediatrics.

In July 1768, William **Heberdon** presented the first clinical description of angina pectoris, in a paper entitled "*Some Account of a Disorder of the Breast*", which he delivered before the Royal College of Physicians in London. In 1785, William **Withering** described a new treatment for dropsy in "*An Account of the Foxglove*", characterizing the use of digitalis leaf for the first time.

And Leopold **Auenbrugger** von Auenbrugg, a Viennese physician published a short treatise: "*Inventum Novum*" (a new invention), describing the innovative technique of chest percussion. As a child Auenbrugger had observed his father, a wine merchant, thumping the sides of barrels to establish the level of potable liquid in the cask. From this it was but a brief leap of ingenuity to employ the method for pleural effusions.

Not all medical discoveries during Mozart's time were respected or admired. Take the case of another Viennese physician, Friederich Anton **Mesmer**. He had established the "Magnetic Institute" of Paris, with support from Louis XVI and Marie Antoinette (she went head over heels for it). Mesmer believed that he possessed occult powers, and he frequently employed hypnotism, astrology, and "magic wands" to achieve cures. One of his more prominent patients was General Lafayette, who fortunately escaped iatrogenic harm in time to assist our fledgling country in its difficult parturition. Eventually, the French Medical Society ousted Mesmer from the country, although his name has survived through the centuries, a "mesmerizing" mountebank in the history of medicine.

Finally, we must note the story of the two **Hunter** brothers, William and John, both of whom graced the Mozart period. William, the elder, was an obstetrician, teacher, and author who, among many other accomplishments, wrote "*The Anatomy of the Human Gravid Uterus*", an anatomic monograph that has rarely been excelled. William had introduced cadaveric dissection to Great Britain and was for years Professor of Anatomy at the Royal Academy. He developed the modern method of arterial injection of embalming fluid in order to preserve bodies for burial. (His brother John utilized the technique to embalm the body of a Mrs. Martin Van Butchell. In her will, Mrs. Butchell had specified that her husband Martin would inherit a vast estate as long as her body remained above ground. The husband complied, placing Mrs. Butchell's preserved remains in a glass-lidded case in their sitting room, for all to visit.)

You may recall that John Hunter was the unfortunate victim of his own imprudence. In a mistaken attempt to demonstrate that gonorrhea and syphilis were the same disease, he inoculated himself with material from a chancre. Years later he died of luetic complications, without the "joys" of acquisition.

In 8 AD, the Roman poet Ovid wrote a famous love poem: *Metamorphoses*. His story concerned Sipylus, the eldest son of Niobe, who lived near - and was named for - Mount Sipylus in Asia Minor. In some versions of Ovid's poem, Sipylus was spelled **Siphylus**.

In 1530, Girolamo Fracastoro, a physician from Verona, composed a poem about a luckless shepherd who had contracted a dreaded sexually transmitted disease. Fracastoro, borrowing the shepherd's name from Ovid, called his protagonist Syphilus. The title of his poem was "*Syphilis sive morbus Gallicus*". Translated it becomes: "Syphilis, or the French Disease."

Thus the sexually transmitted disease **syphilis** was, so to speak, conceived.

Model of a Modern Major-General

The last of the Stuart monarchs was Queen Anne who ruled England from 1702 to 1714. During this period King Charles II of Spain died, leaving no heir to his throne. Louis XIV of France immediately declared his grandson Philip to be the new King of Spain. This decree incensed the British government, which then formed a coalition with the Dutch Republic, the Holy Roman Emperor, Prussia, and Portugal. Their union was known as the Grand Alliance. They launched a war to unseat Philip V from his Spanish throne, a campaign that lasted 13 years. The war was variously known as "The War of the Spanish Succession" or "Queen Anne's War." In North America, it was called the second "French and Indian War."

Although the Duke of Marlborough, John Churchill (distinguished ancestor of Sir Winston Churchill), conducted a superb military campaign against both France and Spain, there were many in England who criticized his strategy and questioned the Queen's policy. One rather obscure man, however, rose passionately to her defense.

His name was Thomas Dover. He came from Bristol, was an accomplished seaman, and had acquired a surfeit of military theory from his father who had been a Royalist cavalry officer. Parenthetically, Thomas was also a physician. Educated at both Oxford and Cambridge, he had subsequently served an apprenticeship under Thomas Sydenham, "The English Hippocrates".

(**Sydenham's chorea**, a neurologic disorder consisting of involuntary movements of the arms, trunk, and legs, associated with gait disturbances and dysarthria, is usually observed in young women, and classically results from acute rheumatic fever. Sydenham first described it in 1686. In 1944 Dr.T.Duckett **Jones** listed the essential features requisite for a clinical diagnosis of rheumatic fever. Among those characteristics, Sydenham's chorea was listed as a major criterion.)

Sydenham's chorea is also known as **St. Vitus' Dance**. Vitus, a Sicilian youth, was murdered in 303 AD during the tyrannical anti-Christian persecutions of the Emperor Diocletian. The martyred lad subsequently attained sainthood, and statues were erected to honor him. Soon afterward, in cities throughout Europe during the 11th and 12th centuries, a grotesque pattern of behavior developed among his worshipers. On the 15th of each June, which was St. Vitus' Feast Day, throngs of celebrants initiated a craze that consisted of maniacal dancing about his shrines. The undulating dancers attained an absolute frenzy of ecstasy, and often many fainted or developed convulsive seizures. Reasons for this bizarre behavior were not obvious, but St. Vitus and his dancing idolaters eventually became a metaphor for rheumatic chorea. The term *chorea* is borrowed directly from Latin and means: "dance." Its roots may be found in such words as **choreography** and **terpsichorean**.)

Returning to our English protagonist Thomas Dover, in 1708 one could find him actively conducting a general practice from a house that overlooked Bristol Harbor. But he was deeply troubled by Spain's denigration of his queen and the insolent Spanish threats to his beloved England. He could not sit idle and do nothing.

Therefore, he outfitted a galleon, hired expert seamen, and began a three-year voyage, which became the most successful pirate crusade in English history. And in the process, he became the first physician-pirate in the world!

Sailing through Drake's Passage around Cape Horn, Dover's men plundered and sacked the Spanish cities of Ecuador and Chile. Following unprecedented success, he and his crew returned to England carrying vast booty, which he proceeded to share with a grateful monarch.

Then he returned to his medical practice, his new wealth permitting a more leisurely pace, and a grateful nation affording an adequate supply of patients.

Thomas Dover (1660-1742) was not only a successful buccaneer, he was equally famous in medicine for having developed a popular sedative consisting of 10% opium, 10% ipecac, and 80% lactose. It was known as **Dover's Powder**. Today it is hardly remembered.

Queen Anne died in 1714 shortly after the Treaty of Utrecht had ended Spanish hostilities. Her entitlement to posterity - as trifling as it was - is forever obligated to the war that still bears her name. Since she had no children, British rule then passed to the German royal house of Hanover, and King George I, who spoke not one word of English, became the next King of England. In 1917 during World War 1, King George V renamed his royal house **Windsor**, in order to divorce himself completely from his original German lineage.

Queen Anne's Lace, a biennial plant in the parsley family, is not named for the preceding English monarch. Rather it is named for Anne of Bohemia, wife of King Richard II of England, who lived in the 14th century. This plant is actually a wild carrot with bitter, albeit edible, roots that were once used as a mild diuretic. Its taxonomic designation *Daucus carota* is distinguished from our domestic carrot, which is *Daucus carota sativa*.

There is one fascinating addendum to the story of Thomas Dover. In the year 1563, a Spanish explorer discovered three tiny volcanic islands in the southern Pacific, approximately 400 miles west of modern Valparaiso, Chile. The explorer claimed the islands for the Spanish king , and had lived on one of them for several years, stocking the islands with domestic pigs and goats. Then he left the islands forever.

His name was **Juan Fernandez** and the islands were eventually named for him. After he departed, the islands remained uninhabited, used mainly by local fisherman, and migrant seamen who briefly stopped to replenish fresh water and food stores after rounding Cape Horn.

In 1704 a pirate ship made such a layover. Among those buccaneers was a Scottish sailor named Alexander Selkirk. One day the Scotsman offended his captain and the enraged skipper banished Selkirk from the ship, marooning him indefinitely on Mas a Tierra, one of the three islets in the Juan Fernandez chain.

In 1709, Thomas Dover and his crew, returning from their successful Spanish raids, responded to a distress signal, which emanated from Mas a Tierra. They soon discovered the deserted sailor, and brought him back to England.

Shortly thereafter, Daniel Defoe made Selkirk into a folk hero for all ages. Based on Selkirk's true story, Defoe wrote **Robinson Crusoe**.

Eponyms V

Across the Bering Sea, directly facing the Chukchi Peninsula of Siberia, is a promontory known as the Seward Peninsula. On its southern shore, bordering Norton Sound, is a town of approximately 2500 Inuit residents. The town is situated near Anvil Creek and, following the discovery of gold in 1898, it became a booming miner's camp with over 20,000 temporary inhabitants. Then they called it "Anvil City."

That is not what we call the town today. In 1849 the British Admiralty decided to chart the waters off the western coast of Alaska. They had directed the H.M.S. Herald to sail through the Bering Straits in order to map the western contour of the land. On arriving at what is now called the Seward Peninsula, the ship's cartographer - not knowing the name of the region - wrote "Cape ? name" onto his preliminary map. Later, as a final blueprint was being completed, a second cartographer, unable to decipher the smudged handwriting, printed "Cape Nome" on the finished draft. The town, henceforth, became **Nome**, Alaska. Thus, sometimes, are names - and eponyms - created. *Sic transit gloria mundi.*

Giovanni Battista **Morgagni** was born in 1682. He graduated the University of Bologna with honors at age 19, having served as pupil under the famous anatomist Antonio Maria Valsalva. At age 30, Morgagni was appointed full Professor of Anatomy at the University of Padua, a post he filled until his death at age 90. Among his scientific contemporaries were Sir Isaac Newton, Edmund Halley, Gabriel Fahrenheit, Francois Marie Voltaire, and Daniel Bernoulli.

Although he was primarily a prosector and anatomist, Morgagni is also remembered for having described several clinical disorders, including the disease we now call **Turner's Syndrome**. He was also the first to describe the features of sudden complete heart block.

It was almost 100 years later (1827) that a paper appeared in The Dublin Hospital Reports entitled: "Cases of Diseases of the Heart Accompanied With Pathologic Observations" by **Robert Adams**. In that paper, sudden death was related to heart block. No mention was made of Morgagni. In 1846, **William Stokes**, who had succeeded his father as Regius Professor of Physic at the Dublin School of Medicine, published a classic paper correlating sudden cardiac arrest with complete heart block. The disorder finally became known as **Stokes-Adams** syndrome. Within recent decades, the discovery of Morgagni's earliest descriptions has led to the more complete eponym: **Stokes-Adams-Morgagni Syndrome**.

Incidentally, **Henry Hubert Turner**, Clinical Professor of Medicine at Oklahoma University, is formally credited with having described Turner's Syndrome. His seminal paper "A Syndrome of Infantilism, Congenital Webbed Neck, and Cubitus Valgus" was published in the November 1938 issue of Endocrinology volume 23:566-574. (The ecchymoses occasionally seen in the flanks of patients with acute hemorrhagic pancreatitis, which is known as the "**Turner's Sign**", was first described in the British Journal of Surgery in January 1920, volume 7, pages 394-5, by English surgeon **George Grey Turner**. He was, as far as I can ascertain, not a relative of Henry Turner.)

John Cheyne (pronounced chay-nee) was another of those exciting and celebrated physicians who comprised "the Dublin School of Medicine". He had studied medicine under Sir Charles Bell (of **Bell's Palsy** fame) at the University of Edinburgh. Subsequently Cheyne became attending physician at Meath Hospital and the first Professor of Medicine at the Royal College of Medicine at Dublin. In The Dublin Hospital Reports Volume two, pages 216-223 (1818) the following article appeared: "*A Case of Apoplexy in Which the Fleshy Part of the Heart was Converted to Fat*". This paper described periodic respirations for the first time. In 1854, William Stokes (see above) verified and extended those observations. We now refer to the phenomenon as **Cheyne-Stokes Respirations**.

There is another story about one of those who formed the famous "Dublin School" of medicine. He was born three years before our Revolutionary War. His father, who owned a successful marble quarry in Kilkenny, Ireland, refused to allow his child to follow that trade. Instead, the boy was sent to study medicine at Dublin and then Edinburgh Universities. Subsequently, he was apprenticed to Sir Astley Cooper (**Cooper's fascia** and **ligament**) in London. Then, at 29 years of age, he was elected president of the Irish College of Surgeons, and became full Professor of Anatomy and Surgery at Dublin University where he remained until his death in 1843. Among his many achievements was a description of the fracture of the distal end of the radius, in which the lower fragment is displaced posteriorly. The man's name was Abraham **Colles** and the eponym, which bears his name, is, of course, **Colles' Fracture**.

There is a footnote to this story. After his death, a post mortem examination of Colles' body was performed by one of his pupils - Robert

Smith. The same Robert Smith who later described a fracture of the distal radius in which the lower end is displaced **anteriorly**. It is often called a **Smith's Fracture** - or a **reverse Colles' fracture**.

Wherever you look, eponyms abound throughout our language. Whether they are macadam highways, pullman Cars, monkey wrenches, tommy guns, good samaritans, tuxedos, magnolias, guppies, or cocker spaniels - they are all named for a person or place. Without them our language would be infinitely leaner, more humdrum, tedious and pedestrian.

The Way of All Flesh

Approximately 60,000 years ago, near what is presently a Kurdish village in northern Iraq, a prehistoric man died and was buried in a cave called Shanidar. He had been a warrior and perhaps had perished during a tribal raid. This young, primeval, combatant was a Neanderthal who had lived at the dawn of human kind - an aboriginal man, uncivilized, unsophisticated, primordial. Yet, someone must have loved him, for in his grave were strewn garlands of hyacinths and daisies. (Palynologists have identified the fossil remnants of their pollen grains within the burial chamber.) The cave at Shanidar marks the earliest known proof of funeral rites.

Neanderthals - officially *Homo sapiens neanderthalensis* - flourished during the paleolithic era (Greek *palaios*: "ancient" + *lithos*: " a stone" - as in **nephrolithiasis** and **lithotripsy**. The **paleolithic** era was the Old Stone Age). The name **Neanderthal** originates from a valley near Dusseldorf, Germany where skeletal remains of *Homo sapiens neanderthalensis* were first discovered. The valley itself was named for an early settler, Joachim **Neander** (German *thal*: "valley" i.e. "Neander's valley").

Anthropologists believe that funeral rites symbolize one of mankind's "rites of passage", which also include birth, marriage and entry into adult society. The ritual observed during each of these ceremonies, serves to assuage man's deepest tribal apprehensions - each society maintaining its own special protective mythology.

The Egyptian **Book of the Dead**, for example, is an elaborate prescription for someone who has just died. It facilitates his/her successful navigation of the underworld. The book is a collection of over 100 texts, translated from ancient Egyptian papyruses, filled with magic spells and hymns to the gods Osiris and Amon-Ra.

It also serves as a textbook for embalmers, describing in detail the techniques for preserving the body - a procedure that often required over 70 days to finish. Ultimately, the corpse was placed within an elaborate coffin displaying an effigy of the deceased carved into the lid. This coffin was known as a **sarcophagus**. According to Pliny the Elder, that term derived from the limestone which lined the coffin, and that completely digested the corpse within a month. (From Greek *sarx*: "flesh" + *phagein*:

"to eat", as in **phagocyte** and **esophagus**. The dead body is literally "eaten" by the coffin.

Pliny the Elder was quite renowned for his thirty seven volume *Natural History*, in which he summarized the existing sciences of his day - astronomy, mathematics, anthropology, pharmacology, and zoology. However, several animals that he described were really mythical and did not exist, and much of his other science was incorrect. Nonetheless, he create the world's first *enkyklios paideia*: "instruction in the circle of arts and sciences" - the first encyclopedia.

Two years after completing his monumental work, Pliny was assigned to command a fleet that guarded the Bay of Naples from marauding pirates. One day he observed a huge cloud overhanging the water. Stepping ashore to investigate the unusual plume, he discovered that the source was Mount Vesuvius itself. It was the morning of August 24, 79 A.D. Shortly thereafter Pompeii, Herculaneum, Stabiae, and Pliny were no more.

The root *sarx* may be found in several common words. For instance, **sarcoma** - a (fleshy) tumor of connective tissue (Greek *oma*: "mass or tumor "), **sarcomere** - the contractile unit of myofibrils, and **sarcoplasm** - the substance in which muscle fibrils are embedded (Greek plasma: "anything formed or molded"). **Sarcoid** is an obscure disorder in which non-caseating granulomas fill the lungs, lymph nodes and spleen producing the "fleshy" appearance of these organs (Greek *oid* from *eides* : " similar to or alike" , i.e. sarcoid is "flesh-like").

Occasionally, even among distinguished intellectuals, one may find a militant muse. He or she will skewer antagonists with rapier wit, a proficiency much admired by some (generally the bystanders), and deplored by others (generally the victims). This clever skill is known as **sarcasm** (from Greek *sarcasmos*, which stems from *sarkazein*: "to tear flesh like a dog"), a succinct Hellenistic metaphor.

(The mythologic **Hellen**, was the son of Deucalion and Pyrrha. His followers, who became the inhabitants of ancient Greece, were named for him. They were called Hellenes, therefore any reference to ancient Greek people, becomes - Hellenistic.)

The Latin root for "flesh" is *carn,* which derives from *carnis*: "meat". A **carnivore** is a meat-eating animal from *carnis* + *vorare*: "to eat" (as in voracious). And the expression "he is the devil **incarnate**" literally means: the devil "in the flesh". **Carnal** knowledge is, well, as Woody Allen once said: "..... the most fun I've ever had without laughing."

The 40 day period from Ash Wednesday to Easter Sunday is known as **Lent** (from the Old English word *lengten* meaning "to lengthen", a reference to that time of the year [springtime] when daylight is growing longer.) The Tuesday preceding Lent is called **Mardi Gras**, literally "fat Tuesday", from the French *mardi*: "Tuesday" and *gros:* "large or big" - so designated for the custom of families eating all meat in their larder, rather than having to throw it out. The act of tossing meat away, known in Latin as *carnem levare,* became our word **carnival**, that festival - renowned in New Orleans - which initiates the Lenten season. Ultimately, its reference to abolishing meat has been forgotten, and carnival has come to mean simply a joyous celebration.

But for the sake of linguistic purity - at the next carnival - dress appropriately. Wear a flesh-colored flower in your button hole.

Wear a **carnation**.

The Flat Mouse

The **platysma myoides** is a thin, flat muscle arising from the pectoral fascia and inserting onto the mandible and **risorius muscle.** Contraction of the platysma draws the corners of the mouth down, as the web of the neck is stretched - a movement often accompanied by outstretched arms with palms up, as one says: "so what?", or "who cares?". **Myoides** means "muscle-like", deriving from Greek *mys*: "muscle" + *eidos*: "resembling". **Platysma** originates from Greek *platys*: "flat or broad".

(The risorius muscle is the smile muscle - from Latin *risus*: "laughter". To ridicule someone is to laugh at them, to act derisively, and to deride them - all stemming from the same root. Facial spasms occurring with tetanus have been called the *risus sardonicus*, a convulsive grin that augurs badly for the unfortunate patient. *Sardonicus*, Latin meaning "of Sardinia", refers to the Homeric legend that a poisonous herb once grew on the island of Sardinia. After eating that herb, a victim invariably died convulsing, with a twisted grin on his face. A sardonic smile is a contorted smirk that conveys bitterness and scorn.)

Platyhelminthes are flatworms (Greek *helmis*: "parasitic worm") and include the pathogenic tapeworms *Taenia saginata* (beef tapeworm), *Taenia solium* (pork tapeworm), *Diphyllobothrium latum* (fish tapeworm), and the *Echinococcus* (dog tapeworm).

Platybasia is a congenital flattening of the occipital skull often causing compression of the medulla and cervical spinal cord.

Platitudes are trite, hackneyed, stereotyped, "flat" and unoriginal remarks. A **plate** is obviously a flat utensil, and a **platform** certainly implies a level or flat surface. ***Plattdeutsch*** is the vernacular language of northern Germany, an area of flat lowlands.

The **Platte** River flows west to east across Nebraska and empties into the Missouri River. It is for most of its 300 miles a broad, flat, shallow body of water. (Plattsburgh, New York which lies across Lake Champlain, a stone's throw from my boyhood home, is **not** flat. It was named after Mr. Zephiniah Platt, a fur trader and land owner.)

A **plat** is a flat diagram or map, which usually illustrates a plot of land. And a **plateau** is elevated and rather flat.

The Duck-billed **Platypus** of Tasmania and eastern Australia displays a broad tail, a snout that resembles a duck's bill, and webbed feet. Its name derives from the latter - Greek *platys* + *pous*: "foot". It is flatfooted.

Plato, the renowned philosopher, was named Aristocles at his birth in 427 B.C. It was much later that he was surnamed Plato, due to his large, flat forehead, as well as his broad expanse of knowledge.

The word **muscle** derives from the Latin *musculus*: "little mouse", which in turn stems from *mus*: "mouse". (A **murine** infection is carried by rodents.) To ancient Romans, contraction of a muscle – such as the Biceps – appeared to resemble little mice running under the skin, therefore the colorful and creative metaphoric name.

In addition to the flat platysma, other muscles were named because of their shape: the **Rhomboid** (a parallelogram with unequal sides), **Deltoid** (triangular, like the fourth Greek letter), **Trapezius** (trapezoidal), **Serratus** (saw-toothed), **Orbicularis** (circular, like an orb), **Pectineal** (comb-like), and **Pyriformis** (pear-shaped) muscles, for example.

The **Digastric** muscle has two bellies, and the **Gastrocnemius** is the "belly" of the leg. (Greek *gaster*: "stomach" + *kneme*: "leg"). The **Lumbricales** reminded some innocent prosector of worms (Latin *lumbricus*: "earthworm"). The **Buccinator** which contracts the cheeks, as when blowing up a balloon or playing the trumpet, is aptly named (Latin *buccinator*: "trumpeter", which ultimately arises from *bucca*: "cheek"). And the **Sartorius** muscle (which flexes the thighs and legs, rotating legs medially and thighs laterally) offers a glimpse into our cultural past. It derives from Latin *sartor*: "tailor" and is responsible for the conventional appearance of these ancient artisans as they worked, thighs and legs flexed, sitting patiently cross-legged on the floor. The affluent clients for whom they toiled, strolled forth subsequently in **sartorial** splendor.

The **Biceps**, **Triceps**, and **Quadriceps** muscles owe their origin to having two, three, or four heads (Latin - *bi*, *tri*, and *quadri* + *caput*: "head").

Finally there are the **sphincters** that control the egress of assorted body fluids from the stomach, biliary ducts, rectum, bladder, etc. The name sphincter originates with that renowned beast of Greek mythology, the **Sphinx**, a chimeric ogre having the body of a lion and head of a woman. The Sphinx was gifted to the city of Thebes by the goddess Hera. There it lay in wait at the front gates, asking each traveler to solve an enigmatic riddle, before he or she would be permitted to enter the city: "What moves on four legs in the morning, two at noon, and three in the evening?" Failure to respond correctly led to a swift death by strangulation. One person, the young Oedipus, correctly responded: "The answer is man who crawls at birth, walks on two legs in adulthood, but must use a cane in old age". The Sphinx was said to have become so enraged at this correct response that it throttled itself to death. Thus we have the origin of sphincter, circular muscles that squeeze tightly at the appropriate time (we hope).

If they fail, just contract the platysma, shrug, and say: *"C'est la vie"*.

Caucasians and Cynics

Colchis was an ancient country located south of the Caucasus Mountains in what is now the independent state of Georgia, formerly of the U.S.S.R. It was in these Caucasus Mountains that Zeus chained Prometheus for having given man fire. And it was also in those craggy peaks that a human skull was once discovered.

The skull was prehistoric but quite well preserved, and it was sent to a scientist for careful study. His name was Johann Friedrich Blumenbach, and he is considered the father of physical anthropology. He was the first man to suggest that humans might be evaluated through comparative anatomy. And he was first to classify human subspecies (or "races") by anthropometric measurements of their skulls.

Based on those measurements, he suggested that there were five families of man: brown (Malaysians), red (American Indians), yellow (Mongols), black (Ethiopians), and white. The last he named **Caucasian**, because the most perfect example of its skull had come from the Caucasus Mountains.

Unfortunately, although Blumenbach did not intend it, his theory has subsidized centuries of bigots who have used it to advance the dogma of racial inferiority - from the ignominy of American slavery - to the perfidy of the Holocaust. He also inadvertently provided physicians with their most consecrated pomposity - heard at almost every case presentation - "A well-developed, well-nourished Caucasian....". And lest we not forget, the tedious drone of the police dispatcher who also uses the same cliché: "Male Caucasian, five foot eight,165 pounds...."

In addition to providing the romantic backdrop for the adventure of the Golden Fleece, Colchis is noted for a native flower, a relative of the hyacinth and lily, which blooms in the fall. It is named for its place of origin: *Colchicum Autumnale*. The plant conceals underground bulbs that produce a remarkable chemical. In 1763,von Storck promoted this chemical for the treatment of gout, calling it **colchicum**. Ben Franklin used it himself, and introduced it into the United States. In 1820 it was purified, and the drug produced was named **colchicine**.

Early physicians believed that gout was caused by specific humors (liquids), which trickle out of the body, drop by drop. The Latin for "drop" is <u>*gutta*</u>, from which <u>gout</u> ultimately evololved.. <u>*Gutta*</u> also gave us "**<u>gtts</u>**" (drops) as a prescriptive term.

In 1542 a professor of medicine at Tubingen, who was also a renowned botanist, described and named a lovely new plant. It grew from 18 to 60 inches in height and displayed purple, bell-shaped flowers. The professor's name was <u>Leonhard Fuchs</u>, for whom the **Fuchsia** was named (as well as the purple dye known as **basic fuchsin**). The plant, which Fuchs himself named, is called *Digitalis purpurea.*

<u>Digitalis</u> owes its genus name to the finger-like flowers (Latin <u>*digitus*</u>: "finger"). Its purple color gives us the species name. In fact there are 25-30 digitalis plants, each of which belongs to the **Foxglove** family. <u>Foxglove</u> derives from *fox,* which is Old English for "folk", referring to the "little people" (elves and fairies). **Glove** evolved from German <u>*gloche*</u>: "a bell". Therefore, Foxglove meant "fairy bells", implying the shape of the flowers, which are either bells or fingers, depending on your quixotic inclination.

Another plant, a small climbing shrub, flourishes in India. It is a member of the **Dogbane** or *Apocynaceae* family, which includes the Periwinkle and Jasmine. In 1703,a French botanist named Plumier named it <u>*Rauwolfia serpentina*</u> in honor of **Leonhard Rauwolf**, a 16th century German botanist.

In 1931, the powdered root of this plant was first used by Indian physicians for patients with hypertension and psychiatric disorders. However, it wasn't until 1955 that Western physicians began to employ it. Shortly thereafter a purified active drug was extracted from the whole root and named **reserpine.**

<u>Dogbane</u> is derived from the belief that the plant was poisonous to dogs (*bane* - Old English meaning "to wound or kill", as in "It was the bane of my existence"). The Latin genus *Apocynaceae* derives from *apo*: "away", and *cynicus*: "dog-like", which evolved from Greek <u>*kyon*</u>: "dog". That is, something that injures or repels dogs.

The constellation Little Dipper, or Ursa Minor, was originally named <u>*kynosoura*</u>: "dog's tail". The brightest star in that constellation is <u>Polaris</u>, the North Star, carefully observed by generations of wandering navigators searching for home. A **<u>cyno</u>sure** started out as a dog's tail, but now is someone or something that is the center of attention.

Someone who is critical or sarcastic, is often called a **cynic**. He or she carries on a tradition instituted by <u>Diogenes</u> and his philosophic comrades who established the school of <u>Cynics</u> - an allusion to the dog-like snarl, and the curled-up lips - of its contemptuous practitioners.

1942: Paradise Lost

[My friend Dan has finally returned to Germany. On April 29, 1945, the morning of his deliverance from obscenity, he had vowed never to go back. It was a Sunday morning and the muddy heroes of the U.S. 42nd Infantry Division - the Rainbow Division - having fought through battlefields of bloody hell, opened a barbed-wire gate and stood mute in the presence of a satanic nightmare. They had walked into Dachau concentration camp. Danny was waiting there for them. He was 15 years old.]

In 1942 William Wrigley's company entered World War II. His corporation suspended peacetime operations to begin packaging field rations for the U.S. troops. These miniature provisions contained canned meat substitute, compressed graham biscuits, three tablets of sugar, a fruit bar, bullion, soluble coffee, a bar of concentrated chocolate, four cigarettes, and - of course - a stick of gum. The abbreviated meal was known as a "**K-ration**" because it had been developed by the physiologist Ancel **Keys**.

(Ancel Benjamin Keys was Director of the Division of Physiologic Hygiene at the School of Public Health, University of Minnesota. He later became known as the earliest proponent of the dietary cholesterol/saturated fat hypothesis in the etiology of atherosclerosis.)

In 1942 World War II was not going well for us, although it may be hyperbole to suggest that K-rations were in any way responsible. The battle of the Java Sea had ended with five Allied ships sunk. On the peninsula of Bataan, Major General Edward King had surrendered his entire army of 76,000 hollow-eyed, bone-weary men, who were subsequently force-marched to the Japanese P.O.W. camps - the infamous "Bataan Death March" - which left 10,000 dead along the route. The island of Corregidor under command of General Jonathan Wainwright was next to fall, and the battle of the Coral Sea soon followed with loss of the American aircraft carrier Lexington. Later that year the cruiser Juneau went down, killing 700 men, including five young men from the same family - the Sullivan brothers. And General Douglas MacArthur had retreated from the Philippines, promising "I shall return".

It seemed an empty threat.

There were, however, a few bright spots for Americans to cheer about. On April 18, 1942 Colonel James Doolittle left the deck of the carrier Hornet with a squadron of sixteen B-25 airplanes and flew toward Japan. They bombed Tokyo, Kobe, Nagoya, and Osaka. The Japanese were stunned. The location of the launch site mystified them. When asked at a subsequent press conference, a smiling F.D.R. told reporters that the bombers had come "from **Shangri-la**".

President Roosevelt loved that name. In fact he later used it to christen the 134 acre presidential sanctuary in the Catoctin Mountains of Maryland. In 1953 Dwight Eisenhower renamed Roosevelt's Shangri-la. He called it "**Camp David**" in honor of his grandson.

The name Shangri-la had come from a 1933 novel by author James Hilton. The story, "Lost Horizon", told of the mythical Shangri-la, a utopian lamasery located in the towering Himalayas of Tibet. Those who lived there could never age - provided they did not leave. In 1937, Frank Capra produced the Hollywood version starring Ronald Coleman, Sam Jaffee, and Thomas Mitchell.

The word **utopia** was, itself, coined by Sir Thomas More, English statesman, lawyer, poet, and humanist. In the year 1516, he had published an essay entitled "Utopia", in which he outlined a society governed so justly as to ensure total freedom for its citizens. Sir Thomas chose the name Utopia quite carefully. He derived it from the Greek *ou*: "not" + *topos*: "place", that is, "not a place", or "nowhere" - indicating his acerbic skepticism that such a paradise could ever exist.

(In 1535, Sir Thomas refused to sign King Henry VIII's "Act of Supremacy", which declared that the king was the supreme head of the Church of England. More's obdurate defiance ensured his eventual execution - and ultimate sainthood. In 1960 British playwright Robert Bolt retold the tragic story of Sir Thomas More in "A Man For All Seasons".)

In 1872, the English satirist Samuel Butler, best known for his novel "The Way of All Flesh", introduced a variant of the utopian theme. In a novel that mocked his contemporaries, Butler wrote of a country in which any illness was considered criminal, the unborn selected their future parents, and terrorists were thought to be philosophers. Butler entitled his novel *Erewhon* - an anagram for "nowhere" - the English equivalent of Utopia.

1942 was certainly an eventful year. Muhammad Ali, Roger Staubach, Aretha Franklin, and Barbara Streisand were all born that year, and broadway legend George M. Cohan, the original "Yankee Doodle Dandy", died. American cities and towns were blacked out at night. Gasoline, sugar, and tires were rationed, and every American knew at least one soldier, sailor, or marine in some remote, hostile, unpronounceable place.

On January 20 of that year, in the Berlin suburb of Grossen-Wannsee a meeting took place under the chairmanship of Obergruppenfuehrer Reinhard Heydrich, chief of the SD (the **Sicherheitsdienst** or "security service" - the intelligence branch of the S.S. – Hitler's **Schutz Staffel** or "protective forces"). This meeting resulted in the *endlosung*: German for "final solution" - the ultimate answer to the "Jewish problem". This solution took the form of camps with names like Auschwitz, Birkenau, Treblinka, Maidanek, Dachau, and Buchenwald.

[Danny was 14 when the S.S. came to his home. They seized his mother, father and younger brother. No one knows where his family was taken or what ultimately happened to them. A railroad boxcar, crammed with terrified people, transported Dan to his first rendezvous with death. Death's name was Auschwitz, and its chief instrument - the "Angel of Death" - was a physician whose name was Josef Mengele.

As Germany began to lose the war, the S.S. frantically removed all Jewish prisoners from the Polish camps and marched them into Germany. They were desperate to complete the "final solution" before the Nazis were forced to surrender. Fortunately for Danny, the U.S. 42nd Infantry moved faster. They rescued him from Gehenna. They opened the gates of Dachau on that Sunday morning in April 1945.

For 35 years Doctor Dan Fischer practiced family medicine in a small New England town. Day by day he returned to each of his patients a small measure of that which another physician - Josef Mengele - had stolen from medicine and from the civilized world.]

At 03:45 P.M. on December 2, 1942 - under the stands of Stagg Field at the University of Chicago - cadmium rods were cautiously withdrawn from graphite blocks containing uranium. It was just one year after Pearl Harbor, and the world had quietly entered the age of nuclear fission.

Less than three years later pilot Paul Tibbets, the **Enola Gay**, and a 9,000 pound bomb would all rendezvous over the Japanese city of Hiroshima.

In 1942, Utopia was nowhere to be found.

Rose Red and Prussian Blue

Botanists have delegated an assortment of ornamental plants to the order of Roses (*Rosales*). Among them are flowering cherries, mountain ash, hawthorn, roses, and spirea.

The family *Spirea* contains over 100 shrubs indigenous to the temperate zone. The leaves of one of them, *Spirea Ulmaria*, furnishes an extract that has an unpleasant, tart flavor. Researchers for the Bayer company in Germany, were the first to purify this substance and to name it *spiroylige saure*. Its principal ingredient turned out to be **salicylic acid**.

In 1899 Felix Hoffman and Hermann Dreser, chemists who worked for the Bayer Corporation, synthesized an acetylated derivative of salicylic acid from coal tar. They discovered that this substance was analgesic (Greek: *an*: "without" + *algesis*: "a sense of pain") as well as antipyretic (Greek: *anti*: "against" + *pyretos*: "fever").Searching for an appropriate name for the new product, they borrowed an "a" from acetyl, "spir" from *spiroylige saure*, and terminated the word with "in". They called it **aspirin**. The Bayer corporation began marketing aspirin in 1905 and it soon became the world's largest selling over-the-counter remedy.

Shortly afterward, Bayer was purchased by a huge German cartel, the I.G.Farben Industries, which had also established an American subsidiary. Following Germany's loss to the allies in World War I, the American Bayer company was regarded as "spoils of war". The U.S. government confiscated it and sold it to the Sterling Drug Company of New York City, which continues to market "Bayer Aspirin" to this day.

The Sterling Drug Company is also noted for its manufacture of "D-Con", a mouse and rat poison containing **warfarin**. Warfarin is the proprietary name for **coumarin**, an anticoagulant that diminishes clotting factors II, VII ,IX ,and X by interfering with gamma carboxylation of precursor proteins. Coumarin is a chemical that can be recovered from the Tonka bean, a fragrant, almond-shaped bean used in many perfumes, and obtained from several leguminous trees of South America. The Tupi Indians of Brazil call the Tonka bean *cumuru*, from which their Portuguese dictators derived the term *coumarou*. Ultimately the term became coumarin.

In 1924 a hemorrhagic disorder was reported in cattle that had ingested spoiled sweet clover. An investigation revealed that bishydroxycoumarin (**dicumerol**) was present in the clover, and was responsible for the bovine bleeding. In 1948, Karl Paul Link, a biochemist at the University of Wisconsin, synthesized **coumarin**, a more potent congener. He secured a patent on the drug and then named it **warfarin**, an acronym for the Wisconsin Alumni Research Foundation plus coumarin. The age of anticoagulants had dawned for man - as well as rats.

The I.G.Farben Company of Germany is quite renowned for other successes. The company name is an acronym, that derives from *Interessen Gemeinschaft Farbenindustri Aktiengeselschaft.* In German, this translates to "a syndicate of dye industries, incorporated". It is actually one of the world's largest consortiums, and has embraced much more than just dye and chemical enterprises. At one time Farben controlled over 500 companies in 92 countries, and was a signatory to over 2,000 cartel agreements. During World War II, Farben Industries controlled more than 900 chemical factories in Germany, and supplied 85 percent of the explosives and virtually all of the tires that were used by the Nazi army. Annually, it submitted to Hitler's government a bill for over $1 billion dollars. (The term Nazi is also an acronym for *Nationalsozialistiche Deutsche Arbeitpartei*: "The National Socialist German Worker's Party".)

There is another, less well known, aspect to I.G. Farben's diverse operations. In the late 1930's one of their chemical affiliates had fabricated a special gas. It became known as **Zyklon-B**.

The chemical method employed to produce this gas was actually quite ancient and well known. It had been developed much earlier in Prussia, where - in 1704 - a stunning blue chemical pigment was originally created . The world called it **Prussian Blue**, and it is still one of the major tints used in the dye and printing industries today.

Prussian blue is ferric ferrocyanide. Utilizing a similar technique, I.G.Farben patented the process for manufacturing solid crystals of **hydrogen cyanide**, which enabled this very toxic substance to be safely and easily controlled and distributed. **Zyklon-B** was initially exploited as a rodenticide and pesticide. Hitler considered that an appropriate irony, because those crystals ultimately became the decisive instrument for his *endlosung* (the "final solution") - his operation to rid the world of Jewish "rodents".

Between 1941 and 1945 the Nazis undertook a massive, systematic, state-sponsored effort to kill every Jew in Germany and within all Nazi occupied territories. The program was run by the **S.S.** under the direction of Heinrich Himmler, Reinhard Heydrich, and Adolph Eichmann. (The S.S. were distinct from the *Gestapo,* which were

Germany's secret state police - an acronym derived from *Geheime Staatspolizei*)

Seven concentration camps were chosen to conduct methodical genocide: Auschwitz-Birkenau, Treblinka, Belzec, Sobibor, Chelmno, and Stutthof. The method used was quite precise. Prisoners were led to *brausebader*: ("showerbaths"). They were stripped naked and escorted into a communal chamber. The doors were then closed and bolted from the outside.

Next, amethyst-blue crystals of Zyklon-B were dumped into the air shaft. Almost immediately, hydrogen cyanide gas was released by sublimation. **Prussic acid**, as the gas was often called, filled the locked room. (Prussic acid was the original term for hydrogen cyanide since it had originally been derived from Prussian blue.) At a lethal dose of one milligram of cyanide per kilogram of body weight, death came quickly. The trivalent iron atoms within cytochrome oxidase bind tightly to the cyanide ion. Intracellular oxidation is completely incapacitated, oxidative phosphorylation ceases, and the Krebs cycle grinds to a halt. A few grand mal seizures are soon followed by apnea and death.

The arterialized venous blood gave the dead a grotesquely robust facial color, as they were dumped into the crematorium for final disposition.

After World War II, twenty four I.G.Farben executives - who had knowingly participated in these obscenities - were charged with enslavement and mass murder. Their trial represented the first such indictment of businessmen in world history. However, because of mounting anxiety that destruction of Farben Industries might worsen Germany's post-war economy, the case was ultimately dropped. The executives were released.

On December 9,1946 twenty three Nazi doctors were brought before American Military Tribunal Number 1 in Nuremberg, Germany. They were all charged with war crimes as well as crimes against humanity. Among those physicians were university professors, the chief administrative (medical) officer of the Reich Chancellery, the chief of medical services for the armed forces, the head of the institute for military research, and Hitler's own personal physician, Dr. Karl Brandt. Seven physicians were executed and five received life terms.

Physicians are, sadly, not much different from others of our putatively moral and advanced species.

I offer an intriguing example of such a medical paradox. There were two men, associated with World War II, whose names I'm certain most physicians will remember. One was a Frenchman named Jules, the other a German named Hans. They were contemporaries, but on opposite sides of the battle line.

Hans was born in Leipzig where he had received his medical degree. After postgraduate training in bacteriology at Paris and London, he became a lecturer at the Institute of Hygiene in Konigsberg, Germany. For a while Hans had worked directly with August Paul von **Wasserman**, famous for having developed the test that bears his name.

In 1914 Hans discovered the Leptospiral organism that causes **Weil's** Disease: *Leptospira icterhaemorrhagicae.* (**H.Adolph Weil**, 1848-1916, first described the clinical manifestations of this disease in Deutsche Archives Klin. Med.39:209-232,1886.)

Subsequently, during World War One, Hans achieved his lasting fame. He had been stationed on the Balkan Front with the 1st Hungarian Army, and here he had observed an interesting, and novel disorder in a young lieutenant. Hans eventually reported the case in Dtsch.Med.Wochenschr. 42:1535-1536,1916 - referring to it as "spirochetal arthritis".

Later on, Hans was mesmerized by Adolph Hitler, and in 1932 signed an oath of allegiance to become a member of the Nazi Party. Hans received several appointments within Hitler's government and was finally chosen to be the Director of the Health Department for the State of Mecklenburg.

Following the allied victory in 1945, Hans was briefly imprisoned in an American P.O.W. camp. When it was ascertained that he had not been associated with the Nazi extermination camps or any of the human experiments, he was released. In 1969, at age 88, Hans – the Nazi physician - died peacefully at his country home in Hesse.

Jules, on the other hand, was a fifth generation physician born in Rouen, France where his father had been professor of anatomy. After medical school Jules began postgraduate work in neurology, studying under **Landouzy** and **Dejerine**. (In 1884, Louis Theophile Joseph Landouzy and Joseph Dejerine described the facio-scapulo-humeral form of progressive muscular dystrophy known by their mutual eponym.)

After a number of years, Jules became chief of the clinic and director of laboratory services at the famous Salpetriere Hospital in Paris. In 1922 he became the first person to describe a pheochromocytoma of the adrenal medulla.

During World War II Jules was an active resistance fighter in the French underground. He and his eldest son, Jacques, rescued and concealed Allied fliers, and then smuggled them across the border to Spain and freedom.

One night his son Jacques failed to return home. The following day, the S.S. arrested Jules, his wife, and their youngest son. After three months in prison, the three were released on insufficient evidence.

Jacques, however, had been taken to concentration camp Dora (Mittlebau) where he was tortured and executed..

Jules never quite recovered from the loss of his courageous son. In 1952, after several T.I.A.'s he died of congestive cardiac failure.

His full name was **Jules Tinel**, and you may remember the two clinical signs identified with his name. One, distal tingling on percussion over an injured nerve, indicating regeneration. The second, percussion over the wrist with resultant tingling in the distribution of the Median nerve, found in patient's with the Carpal Tunnel syndrome. Each is referred to as **Tinel's Sign**.

Our German physician, **Hans Reiter,** had described the urethritis, arthritis, and conjunctivitis, which identifies the syndrome that bears his eponym - **Reiter's Syndrome**. He is also known for the **Reiter complement fixation test** for syphilis.

Here we find two respected physicians on opposite sides of a geographic border. On two sides of a military contest. On contrasting sides of a moral issue.

It appears that moral issues are not always black and white.

Or rose red and Prussian blue.

Prudence, Porkers, Pesos, and Plants

In ancient Egypt, the Pharaoh was known by five separate and illustrious titles. The foremost of these titles acknowledged his descent from Horus, god of the sky. Horus was an imposing figure who flaunted the head of a falcon and whose eyes were made from the sun and moon.

The Greeks borrowed the Egyptian god Horus, and renamed him Harpocrates. One day **Aphrodite**, goddess of love (known as Venus to the Romans), was discovered *in flagrante delicto* by Harpocrates, who threatened to inform the other Olympian gods of her base impropriety. To silence him, Aphrodite's son, **Cupid**, offered Harpocrates a rose - in fact, it was the first rose ever created. Harpocrates accepted, and this flower came to symbolize discretion, even as Harpocrates became known as the personification of tact.

During the Middle Ages, the royalty of Europe built concealed, sound-proof chambers within their castles. These exclusive rooms permitted highly classified matters to be discussed, without fear of intrusion or discovery. The ceilings of these chambers were adorned with ornately carved roses, in deference to Harpocrates. Private conversations held there were considered to be confidential, since they had been conducted "under the rose" - the origin of the term *sub rosa*.

A **poke** is an antique and almost outdated term for a small sack. Its origin comes from Old French *poque* ("bag"), which also yields the terms **pox** (as in small pox), and **pocket**.

In medieval times it was the custom for peasants to market their wares at local county fairs. Young swine were frequent items presented for sale and, being quite small and easily lost, these squirming shoats were often imprisoned in a pouch, the mouth of which had been securely tied with a rope.

Prospective buyers were loath to untie the bag to inspect its content, for fear that the resident within might escape. Therefore, the purchase was quite often a blind one. Unscrupulous vendors were thus able to readily swindle an ingenuous customer by selling a deformed hog, or - worse yet - a scrawny cat, in the guise of a healthy pig.

If, in the process of **buying a pig in a poke**, the unlucky buyer were accidentally to loosen the string - releasing instead a terrified cat - he would have **let the cat out of the bag**. Rather than having bought himself a fine porker, the poor consumer would find himself left **holding the bag**.

When I was a child, an uncle presented me with *Treasure Island* by Robert Louis Stevenson. As you may recall, the story concerns Jim Hawkins who sails away on the **Hispaniola** and, with the assistance of the marooned, slightly demented Ben Gunn, recovers pirate treasure, which had been buried on the island. Unfortunately, Hawkins runs afoul of the iniquitous, diabolical Long John Silver, he of the one wooden leg and loquacious parrot, that interminably iterates and reiterates: "**pieces of eight!! pieces of eight!!**".

The Spanish (Mexican) dollar was commonly used in the United States until well after the Civil War. At that time it was the equivalent of the U.S. dollar and was composed of <u>eight</u> smaller units, gold coins called **reals** (pronounced ree - als). These coins were stamped with the figure "8", indicating that they were worth 1/8th of a U.S. dollar (12.5 cents). They were thus **pieces of eight**. Americans also knew the real as a **bit**, that is "a bit of the Spanish dollar". One **bit**, or one **real**, equalled 12.5 cents. **Two bits** therefore equaled 25 cents.

As in "shave and a haircut, two bits".

Radicals

Etymology is all about the origin of terms, and the roots from which they arise. The Latin for **root** is *radix*. From it we derive **radical**, the foundation or root of something. In current jargon, radical change involves replacing some root aspect of one's life. (It's ironic that today's "radical" was yesterday's fundamentalist.)

Of course, mathematicians use the radical sign to signify the square root of a number. Roots are also an integral feature of most plants. Occasionally, they are edible and become a dietary staple, such as the succulent **radish**, whose root is admired by many gourmands.

The Greek letter *delta* is the fourth letter of their alphabet, corresponding to our letter "D". *Delta,* in turn, was borrowed from the Phoenician's, whose Semitic tongue may still be recognized in modern Hebrew. The first four letters of the Hebrew alphabet are *aleph, beth, gimel, daleth.* Those of the Greek alphabet are *alpha, beta, gamma, delta.* The similarity is quite striking and furthers the theory that many languages have evolved from an ancestral parent tongue, called Indo-European.

The letter *delta* is shaped like a triangle. A river flowing into a bay or estuary deposits mud and silt as its current slows. This fluvial deposit is most often in the shape of a triangle as well. Therefore, it, too, is called a delta, since it looks like the Greek letter. A muscle that arises from the acromion process and the outer third of the clavicle, inserts onto the lateral shaft of the upper humerus, and abducts the arm, is also somewhat triangular in shape. It is named the Deltoid muscle. (Greek *delta* + *oeides*: "like" - that is, delta-like).

The **acromion** process is at the distal end of the scapular spine. It joins the lateral end of the **clavicle** to form the acromio-clavicular junction - the tip of the shoulder. (Acromion - Greek *akros*: "tip, end, or point" + *omos*: "the shoulder"). **Acrocyanosis** is bluish discoloration of the tips of the fingers. **Acromegaly** is enlargement of the distal appendages. (Greek *akros* + *megalo:* "large" - as in megalomania or megalocyte.) An **acrobat** walks on his tiptoes. (Greek *akros* + *banein*: "to walk") And an **acronym** (*akros* + *onym :* "name") is a word constructed from the tips or first letters of a phrase - such as **radar** from radio detection and ranging, or **laser** from light amplification by stimulated emission of radiation. Also,

quasars, which are quasi-stellar objects - remote galaxies at the edge of time.

Governments are geniuses at manufacturing acronyms, as are most military institutions. The recently concluded **NAFTA** Treaty (North American Free Trade Agreement), **NATO** (North Atlantic Treaty Organization), and **UNESCO** (United Nations Educational, Scientific,and Cultural Organization) are but three examples. During World War II a woman might have become a **WAC** (Women's Army Corps), a member of the **WAVES** (Women Appointed for Voluntary Emergency Service), or gone **AWOL** (Absent Without Leave). Worse yet one might have been assigned to **CINCPAC** (Commander in Chief, Pacific). Americans abhorred the German **GESTAPO** (Geheime Staatpolizei: "secret state police"), and our gallant bomber pilots tried desperately to avoid the **flak** exploding around their airplanes (German - *fliegerabwehrkanone*: "bursting antiaircraft fire"). Contemporary pilots are quite familiar with the Russian **MIG** planes, an acronym for the aircraft's designers Artem Mikoyan and Mikhail Gurevich.

One may belong to **CORE** (Congress of Racial Equality) or to **NOW** (National Organization of Women). One may travel to **PAKISTAN**, which was originally composed of Punjab, Afghan provinces, Kashmir, Sind, and Baluchistan. (Pakistan has a double meaning since it also means "holy country" in its native language Urdu.) One may fly **QUANTAS** Airlines (Queensland and Northern Territories Aerial Services) from Australia to Italy and rent a new **FIAT** car to explore the countryside (Fabrica Italiana Automobili Turini - an acronym for the manufacturer, which is located in Turin).

The world of computers has dazzled us with its acronymic concoctions. **BASIC**, a simple programming language, represents Beginners All-purpose Symbolic Instruction Code. **COBOL**, another programming tool, means Common Business-Oriented Language. **GIGO**, a term with which you may be familiar, means "garbage In, garbage out". The most recent innovation refers to the appearance of text on a computer monitor. It is wysiwyg - pronounced "**wizzywig**", and it means: "What You See Is What You Get".

The clavicle articulates laterally with the acromion process and medially with the **manubrium sterni**. The name **clavicle** originates from the Latin *clavicula*: "little key", which in turn derives from *clavis*: "a key". Obviously some ingenuous early prosector thought it looked like something that unlocks doors.

The Latin word *clavis* (key) - as in clavicle - may be encountered in several verbal disguises. A **conclave** refers to a delegation of Cardinals who have been charged with electing a new Pope. These men are confined to a room within the Vatican and locked in with a key from the outside. (Latin *con* : "with" + *clavis*: "key").

An **enclave** refers to an area of land that is completely enclosed within a foreign territory - as West Berlin was inside of East Germany, during the good old days. (French *enclaver*: "enclosed" from Latin: *in* + *clavis*). On the map an enclave resembles a key fitting into a lock.

In 1722, J.S.Bach wrote "The Well-Tempered Clavier", a set of 48 preludes and fugues for the 17th century instrument the **clavichord**. *Clavier* is French for "keyboard". The clavichord succeeded the harpsichord and ultimately led to the invention of the piano. That instrument was originally called the ***pianoforte*** by its inventor, Bartolomeo Cristofori of Padua. This name derives from the Italian *piano e forte*: "soft and loud" - since the keys could be struck softly or loudly using the foot pedals. The ***piano*** endured, but the forte was eventually dropped.)

Latin: *clavis* finally evolved into French: *clef* , bequeathing those friendly signs at the beginning of sheet music, the C, G, and F clefs, which are the keys to the music.

Finally, the French term for a novel whose characters are thinly-veiled parodies of real people is *roman a clef* - a novel with a key.

A **fugue** is a musical composition in which successive melodic themes are repeated in contrapuntal fashion. It derives from Latin *fugere*: "to flee", as in **fugitive**. In a fugue, the serial melodies seem to flee from each other (or chase each other depending on your perspective). In psychiatry a fugue state is one of amnesia - a state in which memory seems to "have fled the intellect".

All of which should prove radical to the discerning mind.

Namesakes

In 1610 the survivors of the decimated Jamestown colony left home and sailed down the James River, heading for the Chesapeake Bay and an anticipated return to England. En route they met the frigate Virginia captained by Sir Thomas West, the 12th baron De La Warr. He persuaded them to return to Jamestown with him, and later became the first governor of the Virginia colony.

Still later, Sir Thomas was assigned to posterity, since both the Bay of **Delaware** and its sovereign state were named after him.

Names of places and things make a fascinating study. **Pennsylvania**, next door to Delaware, was named for William Penn. It is literally: "Penn's **woods**" (Latin - *sylvania*: "wooded land"). **Florida** was named by Ponce de Leon for Easter Sunday, 1513, the day he landed there. He called it *Pascua* (Spanish: "Easter") *florida* (Spanish: "flowering"), that is, "flowering Easter". The "Easter" part was dropped later, leaving merely Florida.

Some of our states were named for English royalty - **New York** and the **Carolinas**, for example, are named respectively for the Duke of York and King Charles 1. (His Latinized name was Carolus.) **Maryland** was named for Queen Henrietta Maria, wife of King Charles.

Most of our state names came to us through the courtesy of our Native Americans. **Massachusetts**, the **Dakotas**, **Michigan**, **Wisconsin**, **Minnesota**, **Mississippi**, **Missouri**, **Nebraska**, **Alabama, Illinois**, **Alaska** - each derive from the language of the Sioux, the Chippewa, the Algonquin, the Iroquois, the Navajo, the Eskimo, the Choctaw, and others.

New Jersey deserves some special attention. It is named for the Isle of Jersey, which is the southernmost and the largest of the English Channel Islands. That island lies approximately 80 miles south of Great Britain and 12 miles west of France. In the 1st century BC, it was conquered by Julius Caesar and subsequently named **Caesaria**. Linguistic evolution over the centuries has gradually altered the name to its present form **Jersey**.

In 1664, the Duke of York granted John Berkeley and Sir George Carteret (former governor of the Isle of Jersey) a charter to establish a colony in the New World, named after the Isle of Jersey. It was to be known as *Nova Caesaria*, and was located south of New York and east of

Pennsylvania. Nova Caesaria soon translated to **New Jersey**, thus adding an occult Roman flavor to our eclectic country.

The Isle of Jersey has exported much more than its name to the New World. A breed of cattle known as Jerseys comes from its rocky shores - as does another, more brown and white cow, from its sister island **Guernsey**. (**Herefords** emigrated from Herefordshire county in England - and are likely to be referred to as "heffers" where I come from.)

In addition to a thriving cattle industry, the Isle of Jersey is famous for exporting a knitted tunic made from wool. This soft garment, invented in the 15th century, absorbs sea spray without feeling uncomfortably wet, and has become the favorite wear of sailors and fisherman. Ultimately it has become known as a "**jersey**", currently the almost exclusive property of football teams. (**T-shirts**, on the other hand, are named for their shape. When unfolded and laid flat - they actually look like the letter "T".)

Incidentally, there was another **Caesaria** founded by those energetic Romans. This one was in Spain and, as was previously explained, it's name also evolved into one with a more local flavor. It is now called **Jerez.** The people in this town make a savory wine, slightly dry to creamy sweet, with a 40 proof label. The English found Jerez difficult to pronounce, so they called the product : **Sherry**.

Most automobiles are also eponymous - titled in more than one way, as it were. The **Buick**, for instance, is named for a plumber who designed the car: David Buick (1855-1929). He was soon muscled out of his own company and died obscurely and quite destitute, a trade school clerk.

I'm certain you also know that Louis Chevrolet designed the Chevrolet, that the **Chrysler** was named for company founder Walter P. Chrysler, and that **Ford** was invented by founder and owner Henry Ford. But did you know that Ransom Eli Olds built the Oldsmobile in 1899? Or that the **Cadillac** is named for Sieur Antoine de la Mothe Cadillac, who was the founder of Detroit (1701) - as well as once governor of Louisiana (1711-1716)?

The **Rolls-Royce** was invented by engineer Sir Henry **Royce** and promoted by a daring soldier of fortune, Charles Stewart **Rolls**, a 19th century "Evel Knievel". Rolls was an auto racer and stunt pilot, and the first Englishman to die in an airplane accident.

Lastly, a new automobile was introduced in 1901 by the German automaker, Gottlieb Daimler. An Austrian consul, Emil Jellinek, agreed to purchase and to distribute Daimler's entire stock of 36 automobiles that were produced that year. There was one precondition: Daimler must rename the entire division of those vehicles after Herr Jellinek's 11-year-old daughter.

Her name was **Mercedes**.

Leo

It was on a midnight shift during the first month of my internship that Leo walked into my life. He entered the emergency room of our city hospital coughing and spitting up blood.

Between deep gasps, he informed us that he was a longshoreman working on the Jersey docks and that several hours earlier, while unloading kegs of nails, a barrel had slipped through his burly arms and jammed itself into his groin. A few nails were protruding from the lower end of the keg and had deeply pierced his left inguinal region. He bore the fresh gashes to prove it. Several hours later he had experienced a lancinating pain in his right chest, so severe that he could not breathe deeply, and he coughed up blood. To substantiate his story, he promptly spat a tablespoon of fresh blood onto the emergency room floor. I later learned that Leo could repeat this performance virtually on command.

A few hours after his admission for suspected pulmonary embolism, I began to harbor suspicions. Leo resembled an orangutan. He was stout, heavily muscled, quite ugly, and his body was covered with the thickest hair I had ever seen. His arms were three times the width of mine. I tried to advance an 18 gauge needle into his antecubital vein, in order to initiate heparin therapy. The arm was so heavily muscled that I found no vein. Leo showed me precisely where the vein was and, covering my hand with his massive paw, guided the syringe to its vascular destination. Denmark began to reek ever so slightly.

Several days after alerting the Jersey City Police, we learned that Leo was wanted on a narcotics charge. It took almost three weeks, however, to convince them that he did not have tuberculosis - indeed that he was not "sick" at all. Eventually they dragged him out of the hospital kicking, biting, coughing blood, and screaming epithets. He threatened to return and kill all of us. My senior resident, Paul, did not sleep for two months. I believe he still occasionally wakens in a cold sweat dreaming of that muscular little anthropoid.

A number of months later, Dr. John Chapman of Iowa State University Medical School published a paper in J.A.M.A. It was entitled: "Peregrinating Problem Patient: The Munchausen Syndrome." That article dealt with my patient Leo - a man who for years had made his living from hemoptysis (site of origin never determined) and one who had submitted himself willingly to invasive medical procedures of unbelievable number, variety, and hazard - a psychopathic personality who had undergone several inferior vena cava ligations, astonishing each successive surgeon who, in turn, discovered his predecessor's sutures. Traveling restlessly back and forth across this nation, Leo always found refuge in hospitals. There he discovered clean sheets, warm food, shelter, and tender care. Altogether, he visited over 100 of them. Leo became famous enough, in fact, to grace the cover of Time magazine.

Karl Friedrich Hieronymus Freiherr von **Munchausen** (1720-1797) was a German officer who had once served with the Russian Cavalry in the 1739 war against the Ottoman Turks. After retiring from the military he settled in the town of Bodenwerder, Germany and gained considerable fame as a story teller. He frequently enlarged and embroidered his tales of daring, all of which were in the mode of Paul Bunyon and his famous Babe.

In 1785, Rudolph Erich Raspe published an account of those magnificent fables in a book entitled: "Baron Munchausen's Narrative of His Marvellous Travels and Campaigns in Russia". A "**Munchausen**" soon came to be synonymous with bravado, affectation, intemperance, and hyperbole.

In a Lancet article (1:339,1951), Dr. Richard Asher published the first description of a malingerer who feigned catastrophic illnesses. Asher coined the term "Munchausen's Syndrome". Six years later I met the doyen of all Munchausen's, the sovereign monarch of medical misinformation. My friend Leo.

To **peregrinate** is "to meander" and emerges from Latin *peregrinus*: "wanderer". The magnificent, endangered Peregrine Falcon - *Falco peregrinus* - was likewise named, for its wandering migratory habits. *Falco* stems from Latin *falx*: "sickle-shaped" and refers to the anatomy of this raptor's claws. (The **falx cerebri** and the **falciform ligament** of the liver are both sickle-shaped.) In ecclesiastical Latin *peregrinus* eventually became *pelegrinus* as an "r" changed to an "l". Much later, in Old English, *pelegrinus* became **pelegrim** - and finally **pilgrim**: "those who travel or wander".

In the 16th century, Queen Elizabeth I reached an accord with the Vatican, and the fledgling Church of England ventured forth, free from Catholic domination. Nonetheless, certain papal influences remained within the English Church. A reform coalition was therefore initiated to "purify" the Church of England against any remnants of "popery". This movement was known as “Puritanism“. A small but extremely fanatic element within that congregation called themselves the English Separatist Church. These parishioners soon lost favor with the majority, and experienced severe persecution.

Initially they escaped to Leyden, Holland, but shortly thereafter elected to pursue a more emancipated existence in the New World. After contracting with a London company to finance the trip, 78 men and 24 women set sail from Southampton, England on a ship named Mayflower. Sixty six days later - November 21,1620 - they landed on Cape Cod in what is now Provincetown, Massachusetts. Later they moved inland to a place which they named **Plymouth**.

These people soon became known as the **pilgrims**. The wanderers. The foreigners.

Parenthetically, they named their new home **Plymouth** in honor of their original home in Plymouth, England - that, in turn, had been so named because it sits at the junction of the Plym and Tamar rivers - at the mouth of the Plym.

A Chemistry Lesson

In November 333 BC Alexander the Great marched triumphantly into the conquered Egyptian city of Memphis, and was crowned Pharaoh. Thus began the circuitous origin of the term **amino** acid.

The principal god of the Egyptians was Ammon or Amon-Ra. It was customary for the Greeks to support local religious custom among their captives. Accordingly, a temple to Ammon and Zeus (supreme god of the Greeks) was constructed in the North African desert .

Desert nights were usually quite cold, therefore visitors to the temple were forced to light a fire in the temple for warmth. Since trees are scarce in desert habitats, the travelers utilized the only fuel readily available – dried camel dung – similar to the buffalo "chips" used by our early Western pioneers. Over many years, the acrid, white smoke deposited a dry, crusty powder on the temple ceiling. This caked material came to be known as *sal ammoniac*, Latin for "the salt of Ammon".

In 1774, Joseph Priestley, a Unitarian minister, friend of Benjamin Franklin, and an amateur chemist, discovered an extraordinarily pungent gas, which emerged when he treated sal ammoniac with an acid. He named the gas **ammonia**, from the parent compound. (Priestley would soon discover another gas that would ensure his fame - oxygen.)

Ammonia (NH_3) combines readily with many chemicals, and its combining form (NH_2) is known as an **amine** group. All **amino acids** are composed of this chemical unit, and since all proteins are made of amino acid sequences - and we are all largely made of proteins - each of us carries within us vestiges of the ancient Egyptian god Ammon.

An **azo** group refers to a chemical sequence containing nitrogen, particularly N-N. Antoine Lavoisier had inadvertently coined the term while conducting experiments on oxygen. He had started a fire within a closed container. When the fire had died out (due to depletion of O_2), he found that the remaining gas within the container would not support life. He, therefore, termed the residual gaseous substance **azoe**, from Greek *a* "not"+ *zoe*: "life". Later it was discovered that this residual gas was actually **nitrogen**, however, Lavoisier's original designation perseveres in the chemical nomenclature: "azo".

The word **acid** entered our language through the Latin <u>acere</u>: "to be sour", the adjective of which is <u>acidus</u>: "sharp,or sour". <u>Acere</u> also evolved into yet another term - *acetum*: "vinegar", the acrid taste of which originates from **acetic acid**, a phrase you should immediately recognize as the height of redundancy. As Latin developed into French, *acere* became *aigre*, which also means "sour". *Vin aigre* means "sour wine" - or - vinegar.

The Latin *acere* (sour or sharp) was itself derived from *acus*: "needle" as in the term **acupuncture**. One with clinical **acumen** is a "sharp" physician, and one with **acute** hearing has very "sharp" auscultatory skills. (An **acute** angle is quite pointed, and a patient with an **acute** abdomen has a stabbing bellyache.)

The opposite of an acid, which yields a proton, is an alkali, which provides a complementary electron. The origin of the term **alkali** is somewhat convoluted. Ancient people did not have soap. The closest they came to such cleansers was a combination of certain oils mixed with an abrasive material. The abrasive was prepared by burning certain grasses and wood, placing the ashes into a pot of water, pouring off the undissolved solids, and boiling the remaining mixture. After the water had completely evaporated, the residual ashes were removed from the pot, heated together with oils, and this unique compound was then used for cleaning. The Arabs called the ashes *al quili*: "plant ash" - which ultimately became alkali.

Since the ashes remained within the cooking utensil, they were also referred to as "pot ashes" - or simply **potash**. In 1807 a British chemist, Sir Humphry Davy, passed an electric current through molten potash and discovered a new metallic element. He named the material for its source, calling it **potassium**. Much later other scientists decided to provide the element with a more elegant Latinized name. They named it **kalium**, deriving that term from the word alkali. This not only gave us a bogus Latin name, but also provided science with a distinguishing chemical signature: "**K^+**". (Incidentally, potash is principally composed of potassium hydroxide.)

In 1808 Davy once again made an elemental discovery. He heated limestone and recovered a metal that he promptly named **calcium** from the Latin word for limestone - *calx*. (Limestone is mainly $CaCO_3$. Heating it drives off CO_2, leaving residual calcium.)

A small stone, or pebble, in ancient Rome was called a *calculus*. During those early times, people reckoned arithmetically by using a counting board, known as an **abax**. By stringing pebbles into rows and sliding the stones back and forth as one counted, one could easily add and subtract large numbers. The abax is now known as an **abacus**, however, the mathematics is performed by **calculators**. In 1684 two friendly scientific rivals simultaneously developed a new mathematical system. Sir Isaac **Newton** and Gottfried Wilhelm **Leibniz** each separately published the method. It was called the **calculus**.

Their friendship subsequently dissolved .

A yet more primitive method of counting involves the use of fingers (and toes). Since the Latin for this part of one's anatomy is known as a *digitus*, the numbers derived are called digits. Today we have something known as a **digital calculator**, which incorporates neither fingers nor stones.

A kidney stone is logically called a calculus. And certain metabolic states - such as primary hyperoxaluria - cause a disorder known as **nephrocalcinosis**. However, true to the inconsistencies of language, a stone within the renal pelvis or ureter is known as nephro- or uretero - **lithiasis** (Greek *lithos*: "stone"), and the surgery to remove it is called a **lithotomy** (Greek *tome*: "a cutting", as in **anatomy** - "to cut up".)

A **lithograph** is a picture (Greek *graphein*: "to write") created by designs that are cut into flat stones (or currently onto flat metal plates).And the archaeological periods known as the Stone Ages are referred to as the **Paleolithic**, **Mesolithic**, and **Neolithic** eras (*palaios* : Greek - "ancient", *mesos*: "middle", and *neos*: "new"). **Megaliths** are giant (Greek *megas*: "huge") stones used in ancient monuments, such as those on Easter Island or at Stonehenge. A **monolith** (Greek ***monos*** : "single, one") is a statue or obelisk carved from one stone. (A monolithic philosophy is metaphorically one, which has a uniform, inflexible character.)

The **os calcis** or **calcaneus** is, of course, the heel bone - named for its resemblance to a large stone. When heel spurs develop, perhaps we should refer to them as calculi of the calcis.

Wine was known as *methy* in ancient Greece. Wood was called *hyle*. Therefore, wood alcohol (or wine) was known as *methy* +*hyle* or **methyl** (CH_3 groups). Today we clearly understand that wood alcohol is not safe to drink. The ancients, however, had another method of protection against the toxic effects of their libations. They trusted in the deterrent attributes of a lovely purple jewel, which was worn about the neck - or occasionally, molded into a drinking glass. They relied on that enchanted jewel to safeguard them from old John Barleycorn, and they named the precious stone *amethyein* - *a*: "not" + *methyein*: "intoxicated" (derived from *methy*).

We know this jewel as an **amethyst**.

Eponyms VI

In a region known today as Lancaster County, Pennsylvania, there is a river that was known to the Delaware Indians as **Susquehanna** – which translates into: “muddy waters”. The Huron Indians had their name for this river as well, calling it **Kanastoge –** which also translates into: “muddy waters”. The region soon became known as the **Conestoga Valley**. It was noted for two industries. The first, the famous **Conestoga wagon**, was pulled by four to six horses, had a load capacity of six tons, broad wheels that would not easily sink into the mud, and a floor that curved up at each end to prevent contents from shifting. Pioneers emigrating west covered these wagons with white sailcloth, and traveled in long caravans toward their dreams. Seen from a distance, obscured by the tall, waving prairie grass, these wagon trains resembled sailing ships – thus the name **Prairie Schooners**.

The second industry indigenous to the Conestoga region was the manufacture of cigars. Muleskinners, who drove the Conestoga wagons, loved to smoke them. Soon the cigars were nicknamed for the wagons. They were called “**stogies**”.

The naming of American towns, villages and cities makes fascinating study. Many places were named for the indigenous Americans who were native to the region. Towns such as **Des Moines**, Iowa named for the **Moingona** Indian tribe, from which both the river and the city were derived (French: *des Moingon* - “of the Moingona”), **Appomattox**, Virginia (named for a tribe of the Powhatan Indians), **Pawtucket**, Rhode Island (from the language of the Narragansett tribe; it means “falls of water”), **Waco**, Texas (named for the Waco Indians), **Sheboygan**, Wisconsin (from the language of the Potawatami Indian tribe; it means “rumbling waters”), **Kalamazoo**, Michigan (also from Potawatami: “where the waters boil”), **Chicago** , an Algonquin term meaning : “onion or garlic smell”, a reference to nearby fields of wild onions. Also states such as **Nebraska**, **Mississippi**, **Connecticut**, **Alabama**, **Arkansas**, **the Dakotas, Ohio, and Oregon**, all were of Native American origin. In fact, from **Narragansett** to **Napa** our geography is richly endowed with the language and imagery of our original citizens.

Within the elephantine structure of New York City, there exists a borough. In more halcyon days it was the site of a large farm owned by a

Dutchman named Jonas Bronck. When asked where they were going, people would respond: "To the Bronck's". With slight modification in the spelling, the place is now called the **Bronx**.

There is also a section of land located in the southern district of the borough of Brooklyn, New York. Originally, this region was an actual island, separated from Brooklyn by a spit of ocean water. However, as time passed, the sea deposited tons of silt there, ultimately establishing a land connection to the mainland, and making the "island" into a peninsular appendage. The original settlers had discovered innumerable rabbits populating that island. The Latin term for rabbit is *cuniculus*, therefore, the British called these cute, long-eared mammals "cunnies" or "conies". The island became known – you may all ready have guessed - as **Coney Island**.

Many settlements were named for exceptional people who had explored the area, pioneered in its colonization, or were selected for special recognition. **Dallas**, Texas, for example, is named for George Mifflin Dallas who was Vice-President of the United States under James Knox Polk. **New York City**, and **Yorktown**, Va. were each named for the son of King James I of England - the Duke of York - who later reigned as Charles I. (Unfortunately, Charles also presided over the English Civil War and ultimately lost his head over it in 1649.) **Albany**, New York, is named for James, Duke of Albany, who later reigned as James II of England.

Other eponymic communities come quickly to mind: **Cleveland**, Ohio, (for General Moses Cleaveland, who designed the city), **Houston**, Texas (for Sam Houston, president of the short-lived Republic of Texas), **Denver**, Colorado (for J.W. Denver, governor of the Kansas Territory), **Lubbock**, Texas (for Colonel T.S. Lubbock, organizer of the Texas Rangers), and **Raleigh**, North Carolina (for Sir Walter Raleigh), to name just a few. Of course, there's also **Lincoln**, Nebraska, **Madison**, Wisconsin, **Jackson**, Mississippi, and **Monroe**, Louisiana – whose origins I leave to your speculation. However, I believe the state that is the "mother of all eponyms" is Maryland. It excels in titular nepotism, as witness the plethora of names generated by its founding family.

For sixteen years George **Calvert** had been a member of the English House of Commons, a secretary of state and member of the Privy Council. He resigned those positions in 1625 after he had converted to Roman Catholicism. (England's "state" religion was Anglican by this time). Shortly thereafter, the king appointed Calvert to become the first Baron Baltimore with vast land holdings in Ireland. Calvert then established a colony in Newfoundland, which he christened Avalon. Unfortunately the foul weather obliged him to petition King Charles I for another land grant - one with a milder climate.

George Calvert died in 1632 before his request was honored. The charter of Maryland therefore passed to his eldest son Cecilius (Cecil), the 2nd Lord Baltimore. In 1634, Leonard Calvert, Cecil's younger brother, landed on Blakiston Island in the lower Potomac River. This area is now St. Mary's County. Its county seat **Leonardtown** is named for Leonard Calvert, who became the first governor of the colony.

Obviously **Baltimore** County, and **Baltimore** City were named for the Lords Baltimore. **Ann Arundel** County is named for Cecil Calvert's wife, Anne Arundell. Its county seat is **Annapolis** - Anne's city (from Greek *polis*: "city") – and it simultaneously serves as the state capital.

Calvert and **Cecil** Counties are easily identifiable eponyms. **Charles** county is named for Cecil Calvert's and Ann Arundell's son Charles, who was the third Lord Baltimore. (**La Plata** - the county seat of Charles County - is named for silver mines that were found there. From Spanish *plata*: "silver"). **Worcester** County is named for Edward Somerset, sixth Earl of Worcester, who was George Calvert's son-in-law. **Somerset** County is also named for him.

Dorchester County is named for Richard Sackville II, 5th Earl of Dorset, who was a close friend of the Calvert family. (One might note that words ending in "caster" - as in Lancaster, or "chester"- as in Manchester - come from Latin *castrum* : "fort or camp". Thus Dorchester means "Dorset's encampment".)

Caroline County is named for Caroline Calvert, the sister of Frederick Calvert, the sixth Lord Baltimore, and Harford County is named for Henry Harford, Fred Calvert's illegitimate son. **Frederick** County and its county seat are each named for Frederick Calvert, who also finds some distinction as the last proprietor of the Maryland colony.

Regal eponyms also flourish within our otherwise unpretentious state. **Queen Annes, Prince Georges,** and **Kent** Counties derive respectively from England's Queen Anne (1702-1714), her husband-consort Prince George of Denmark, and Edward Augustus the Duke of Kent (Queen Victoria's father). And, of course, **Maryland** itself derives from queen Henrietta Maria, wife of King Charles I.

Three counties bear tribute to Revolutionary War heroes. **Montgomery** County honors General Richard Montgomery who was born, appropriately enough, in Swords, County Dublin, Ireland. In 1773 he emigrated to America and, at the outbreak of the Revolutionary War, was appointed Brigadier-General of the Continental Army. In November 1775 he commanded the expedition that captured Montreal. One month later he was killed during the invasion of Quebec.

Bordering the northeastern perimeter of Montgomery County lies **Howard** County, named for John Eager Howard, soldier of the Continental Army, member of the Continental Congress, Governor of Maryland, and member of the United States Senate. Adjacent to Howard County lies **Carroll** County, named for Charles Carroll, member of the Continental Congress and United States Senator. He was one of four Marylanders who signed The Declaration of Independence, penning the words: "Charles Carroll of Carrollton". He was also a founder of the Baltimore and Ohio Railroad.

Two other counties deserve eponymic recognition. **Washington** County surely requires no explanation. **Garrett** County, on the other hand, may be less readily identified. It is named for John Work Garrett an industrialist, and president of the Baltimore and Ohio Railroad from 1858-1884.

There are two additional counties in Maryland that do not owe their title to the Calverts, or to royalty, or to American heroes, or to the captains of industry. They are **Wicomico** and **Allegany** both of which are obligated to the original Native Americans from whom we have taken so much.

Finally, we return to the original community established by Leonard Calvert. The county we know as **St. Marys**, named for the Virgin Mary by those early colonists - people who had come to this new land seeking religious freedom - driven from their native England by prejudice and cruelty.

They sought spiritual independence for all religions and found it in the new colony of Maryland.

Sometimes we forget that.

Quatrains

The Latin word for "four" is *quattuor*. The prescriptive quater in die - "four times a day" or Q.I.D. - derives from it. The **quadriceps femoris** muscle, the friend of the professional punter, is named for its four heads (Latin - *quadri*: "four" + "ceps" from Latin *caput*: "head").

Quadriplegia (Greek *plege*: "a stroke or paralysis"), and **quadriparous** (Latin *parere*: "to bring forth or deliver") are self-explanatory. *Parere* is also responsible for **parent, parturition,** ante- and post- **partum** and **transparent**.

Quadrigeminy is unfortunately an etymological mistake. It refers to a cardiac rhythm in which every fourth beat is unexpectedly premature, most often an ectopic ventricular beat. However, the term "geminus" itself means: "occurring in pairs or couplets", and derives from Latin *gemini*: "twins". A **bigeminal** rhythm (in which a pair of beats is followed by a pause, then another pair, a pause, etc.) is actually redundant since bigeminy should mean "two twins" or two pairs. (Latin *bi*: "two"). **Trigeminy** (three pairs) and **quadrigeminy** (four pairs) are therefore also misnomers.

(The constellation **Gemini** may be found in the southern sky above and to the left of Orion, easily seen during the winter months. Its two brightest stars are Castor and Pollux, the mythological twins for whom the constellation is named.)

Quartan malaria, caused by *Plasmodium malariae*, is characterized by a high fever that recurs every four days, the result of the protozoa dividing within the red cell, rupturing the cell membrane, and releasing scores of merozoites. (Greek - *meros*: "part" + *zoion*: "animal", i.e. "a part of an animal" - the offspring of asexual plasmodial reproduction One finds the word *meros* in terms such as "centromere" and "telomere". The word **Malaria** itself derives from Italian *mala*: "bad" and *aria*: "air", referring to a primitive belief that the putrid, miasmic vapor rising out of a swamp was the cause of this febrile illness. The ancients were actually very close to the truth - barely missing the true vector *Anopheles,* whose nuptial bed was sheltered within those swamps. (Anopheles stems from Greek *an*: "without" + *opholos*: "use", that is useless - or more properly - harmful.

Typhus, a group of disorders caused by **Rickettsial** organisms, derives from the Greek *typhos*: "smoke, clouds or vapor", a reference to its presumed etiology, a myth analogous to malaria. There are three forms of Typhus. Epidemic Typhus is caused by **Rickettsia prowazekii**, and transmitted by the human louse, **Pediculus humanis**. Endemic typhus, caused by **Rickettsia typhi**, is carried by rodents (thus "Murine" typhus) and transmitted by their fleas. The third form of Typhus is known as "benign" typhus, also called **Brill-Zinsser's Disease**.

Rickettsial organisms owe their genus name to Howard Taylor **Ricketts** an American pathologist who discovered the organism responsible for **Rocky Mountain Spotted Fever** (Rickettsia rickettsiae). Dr.Ricketts later moved to Mexico to investigate a disease known there as **Tabardillo**, which ultimately proved to be Endemic or Murine Typhus. Unfortunately, he contracted the disease and died in 1910 at the age of 39.

Stanislas Joseph Matthias von **Prowazek**, a German zoologist, became interested in those same tiny pleomorphic rods. In 1913 he traveled to Constantinople to study a Typhus epidemic. There he convincingly validated Howard Ricketts' original observations. Unfortunately, Von Prowazek also succumbed to the deadly organisms and died in 1915. He, too, was but 39 years old. The taxonomists have immortalized both men.

"Benign" Typhus is actually a recrudescence of epidemic typhus in patients who have become partially immune to the disease. The infection may remain latent for as long as 70 years after the initial illness. Nathan Brill, a professor of clinical medicine at Columbia University, first described it in 1910. Brill's observations were later confirmed by Hans Zinsser who was professor of bacteriology at that same institution, and the disorder was ultimately named for the two men.

Brill is also remembered for describing the clinical and pathological features of **Gaucher's Disease**, and for first suggesting splenectomy as a treatment for idiopathic thrombocytopenic purpura. Zinnser, pre-eminent in bacteriology for decades, wrote the biomedical classic "Rats, Lice, and History".

(Philippe Charles Ernest **Gaucher**, was a French dermatologist, who first described the disease, which bears his name in 1882. Today, Gaucher's disease is known as a lipid storage disorder caused by a genetic deficiency of glucocerebrosidase.)

The Rickettsioses embrace a number of other well-known disorders, including Rocky Mountain Spotted Fever, Boutonneuse Fever, Rickettsialpox, Scrub Typhus, and Q Fever.

Boutonneuse Fever, known by our French cousins as *Fievre Boutonneuse*, is a disease similar to Rocky Mountain Spotted Fever though much milder, occurring in most Mediterranean countries, Africa and the Middle East. It is heralded by a primary skin lesion, a black spot found at the site of the tick bite, which is known as the *tache noir*. The resemblance to a small buttonhole (French: *boutonniere*) endows the illness with its name.

Scrub Typhus, also known as **Tsutsugamushi Fever**, derives from the Japanese *tstsuga*: "harmful or dangerous" + *mushi*: "insect", a reference to the Trombiculid mites, which transmit the disease.

Q Fever, caused by *Coxiella burnetii* is an unusual Rickettsial infection in that it is not spread by the bite of arthropods. Instead, dried tick feces are inhaled with dust or ingested in milk. The disease puzzled microbiologists and epidemiologists for years, and became known as the "Query" disease, later shortened to **Q** Fever. The organism that causes Q Fever is named for an American bacteriologist, Herald Rea **Cox**, and Noble laureate Frank MacFarlane **Burnet**, who isolated the organism in 1937. (Burnet, an Australian virologist, shared the 1960 Nobel Prize for physiology and medicine with British zoologist Peter Medawar, for discovering that animal embryos may develop immunological tolerance to administered antigens, thus leading the way to transplant procedures.)

The number "four", *quattuor* in Latin, is *tettares* in Greek, from which we derive the combining form **tetra**. In 1948 an antimicrobial substance was obtained from several soil species of the genus Streptomyces. Chemically this antibiotic consists of a four-ring structure, and clinically it is lethal to the Rickettsial family.

Today it remains the drug of choice for treatment of most Rickettsioses.

It is called **Tetracycline**.

Index